GLUTEN ATTACK

Professor David S. Sanders

Vermilion
LONDON

1 3 5 7 9 10 8 6 4 2

Vermilion, an imprint of Ebury Publishing,
20 Vauxhall Bridge Road,
London SW1V 2SA

Vermilion is part of the Penguin Random House group of companies whose
addresses can be found at global.penguinrandomhouse.com

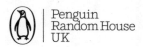

Penguin
Random House
UK

First published by Vermilion in 2016

www.eburypublishing.co.uk

A CIP catalogue record for this book is available from the British Library

ISBN 9781785040160

Printed and bound in Great Britain by Clays Ltd, St Ives PLC

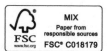

Penguin Random House is committed to a sustainable
future for our business, our readers and our planet.
This book is made from Forest Stewardship Council®
certified paper.

Contents

Continued

Introduction

I am sitting next to a semi-professional athlete by chance. We know nothing of each other's backgrounds or interests. We have time to kill and are making small talk. I ask him about his training schedules and then curiosity gets the better of me. 'What do you think of gluten? Do you avoid it?'

'Gluten, gluten is the devil!' he replies. I smile at the depth of sentiment in his response. My own background is medical: I am a Professor of Medicine and my specialist interest is coeliac disease and thus gluten. For many years I have been seeing patients in clinic who do not have coeliac disease but self-report symptoms related to eating gluten. I have often wondered why, and it has taken me a long time to acknowledge that something may be amiss.

Medicine is complex; it is neither a science nor an art but something in between. This can mean that novel medical concepts may take many years to become accepted practice.

In the course of this book I hope to explore the effects of gluten from a medical perspective and to make sense of what is being reported in the press. I believe there is no doubt something has happened or is happening to society and our relationship to gluten and therefore wheat. I would like to share the unbiased evidence with you and let you make your own mind up.

CHAPTER 1

The world according to Gluten!

Djokovic is not alone!

When Novak Djokovic won again at Wimbledon he ate a small piece of grass as part of his celebration ritual and joked that it was okay as this was 'gluten-free'. By no means is Djokovic alone in his views.

Currently the gluten-free market is outselling all other diet options. Google trends demonstrate a year on year rise in this phenomenon starting around 2004 with gluten-free outselling both low carbohydrate and fat-free diets. The gluten-free industry worldwide is estimated by Reuters to increase from $1.31 billion (2011) to a projected market of $23.9 billion by the year 2020.[1,2]

You Gov (a UK based population survey) reports that 60% of people purchase or consume gluten-free products. This second statistic may be misleading. The recognition commercially of the importance of gluten-free has led to many manufacturers both producing and labelling their goods as gluten-free. Thus we all may purchase gluten-free products without realising it. This does not mean we are making an active choice to be gluten-free. However, there is no doubt that a significant proportion of society has recognised that there is something about gluten that disagrees with them. When delving deeper into the You Gov survey, 10% of households has someone who reports or believes that gluten is bad for them (this work is based on 1,600 representative adults sampled across the UK).[3]

Our centre, the Sheffield Institute of Gluten-Related Disorders (SIGReD), is the largest centre in the United Kingdom and internationally recognised for the work that we have been undertaking dating back to 1996. Our work has encompassed both coeliac disease (more of that later!) and other problems related to eating gluten. In 2013 we published the first population survey of the self-reported effect of gluten from the United Kingdom. We literally went onto the streets of Sheffield and asked more than 1,000 people whether they had symptoms related to eating gluten. Of course it was not the only question we asked them and this study was published after medical peer review in a learned journal.[4] We established that 13% of the population report symptoms when they eat gluten and furthermore 2.9% are on a gluten-free diet of their own choosing. These were individuals who said they had already been tested for coeliac disease or had coeliac disease excluded by their doctors. I must say that this is an important message that I will stress throughout the book:

Rule number 1 of Gluten Attack:

If you have symptoms when you eat gluten please go and see a doctor. Do not place yourself on a gluten-free diet no matter how fed up you may be (even with doctors!). Try to clarify the diagnosis medically once and for all.

If you don't have a medical diagnosis, once you have started a gluten-free diet, you will never really know what it is you are suffering from. A self-imposed gluten-free diet is hard to go back on and has long-term implications. There are many reasons why people have symptoms related to eating gluten as I will describe in subsequent chapters, so getting it right from the beginning will, I hope, help you in the end.

One of the other important findings of our population based study was that people had many and diverse symptoms when they ate gluten, not just gut symptoms, and that these individuals identified an improvement in their overall wellbeing after giving up gluten.

So has any other work been done in this field? I have created a table below that summarises the existing world-wide published surveys available on the subject:

Table 1. International reporting of prevalence of non-coeliac gluten sensitivity

Country	Year	N = the number of people surveyed	% Prevalence in the population surveyed	Further details
USA	2012	5,896	5.9%	Secondary care referrals: Patients referred into the hospital so not a true representation of the size of the problem in society
New Zealand	2012	916	4%	NZ children report gluten avoidance
United States of America	2013	7,798	0.6%	National Health and Nutrition Examination Survey
United Kingdom	2013	1,002	13% or 2.9%	13% report symptoms related to gluten population survey but only 2.9% on GFD
Australia	2014	910	41.2%	Athletes!
Australia	2014	1,184	9.4%	Adult General Population
United States of America	2015	14,701	0.8%	National Health and Nutrition Examination Survey

What this table tells us is that self-reported gluten sensitivity ranges from 0.6% to 41.2% in the published medical literature. It is interesting to note that the 41.2% is something of an outlier and as you can see from the table this specifically relates to athletes while the other studies are population based. This perhaps comes back to what my semi-professional athlete acquaintance told me and reflects or supports what he believes. It would suggest that within athletic and sporting circles gluten is currently viewed with suspicion. Another interesting trend is that all of these studies are very recent, with no data before 2012 or so it seems. So who is driving that agenda? As another medical friend said to me recently, 'I don't see many cases of non-coeliac gluten sensitivity being reported in the developing world!'

Here is the counter argument: non-coeliac gluten sensitivity is driven by the food and gluten-free industry. Your average gluten-free product is four times more expensive than its equivalent counterpart and it is big business.[5] Furthermore this trend is fuelled by celebrity endorsement of the gluten-free way of life. The so called 'lifestylers' or 'free-from lifestylers' who believe that gluten is something inherently worth excluding. If we come back to the Google trends I mentioned earlier and superimpose celebrity endorsement across the timelines (of 2004 to present) it tells an interesting story. In 2006 Oprah Winfrey went on a '21-day cleanse' diet and during this time among other things she gave up gluten. Since that time other celebrities listed on the gluten-free roll call are Gwyneth Paltrow, Victoria Beckham, Rachel Weisz, Michael Douglas and Miley Cyrus. If we then look at the publication of 'anti-gluten books' since 2006 there are many: *The Shocking Truth About Gluten (the brain grain connection)* 2006 (Dr Rodney Ford, New Zealand), *The Gluten Effect* 2009 (Drs Vikki and Richard Petersen, USA), *Wheat Belly* 2011 (William Davis, MD USA), *Grain Brain* 2013 (Dr David Perlmutter, USA), *Serve to Win* 2013 (Novak Djokovic) you could then suggest that a steam-roller effect is occurring against gluten. This has also resulted very recently in controversy with Dr Alan Levinovitz (a doctor of religion and literature from the James Madison University, Virginia, USA) publishing *The Gluten Lie* 2015. This gives an almost diametrically opposed view to the earlier publications and has been described as 'incendiary journalism'. I don't think controversy is a bad thing, but I want to make a point here about differentiating why people avoid gluten. Those people who have recognised that they have symptoms when they eat gluten and may have even noticed that they feel better on a gluten-free diet (bearing in mind rule number one of Gluten Attack on page 2) are very different to someone who simply believes they should not eat gluten or that gluten is somehow harmful.

Rule number 2 of Gluten Attack:

There is no need for everyone to be on a gluten-free diet and if it is a lifestyle choice that you have made then currently it is without proof.

I like history not just because it tells you what has happened but because it also tells you what is going to happen. I believe mankind repeats itself recurrently. When I went back into the medical literature I discovered that there had been three reports that had been forgotten in the mists of time. All three reports (some dating back to the 1970s) describe patients with gut symptoms, typically bloating and diarrhoea. These patients all had coeliac disease carefully excluded by doctors using conventional and accepted medical tests. However, after this the patients all report that their symptoms resolved on a gluten-free diet and that the reintroduction of gluten caused deterioration in their symptoms. At that time the medical debate about the proof or validity of these observations could best be described as 'heated exchanges'. The medical community would not accept that patients could attribute their symptoms to gluten in the absence of coeliac disease. So the earliest reports of what we could now term as non-coeliac gluten sensitivity were discarded by the scientific community. I would suggest that this is evidence that non-coeliac gluten sensitivity may have existed for some time. These historical reports predate any industry or celebrity involvement by decades, though I accept these newer players (industry and celebrity endorsement) may have fuelled the recent interest. However, we must be careful not to ignore or discard our observations again second time round and let medical history repeat itself; this may do society and our patients (in my case) a disservice.[6–11]

The rise and rise of wheat

Where it all begins: 'The Fertile Crescent'

Although mankind may have existed in some progressive form for 2.5 million years it is only in the last 10,000 years that we have been exposed to wheat. Wheat was originally cultivated in the Fertile Crescent (South Western Asia or what is now Turkey, Iraq, Iran, Palestine, Syria and Lebanon) with a farming expansion that lasted from ~9000 BCE to 4000 BCE. So it could be considered that wheat and therefore gluten is a relatively novel introduction to our diet.

In Jared Diamond's (Professor of Geography and Physiology at University of California, Los Angeles) Pulitzer Prize winning book *Guns, Germs and Steel* he reveals a fascinating journey for mankind. For whatever reason compared to the rest of the world the Fertile Crescent created the perfect requirements for cultivation. This allowed humankind to beat the nomadic hunter gatherer trap. For the first time, humans could now cultivate food and did not have to chase food or scour the land looking for it. Humankind could stay in the same place, endure winters and become a farming culture. The first steps towards civilisation. What happens next as a result of this is that larger dwellings of humankind can occur. This of course leads to infection (germs). Many men, women and children died but those who did survive were stronger – an accepted biological concept called 'herd immunity'. So now we have large numbers of hardy men and women with a surplus of food. This inevitably means they can turn their attention to their neighbours and conquest (steel). Thus ruling classes, empires and indeed contemporary civilisation are born. Wheat was at the very heart of our struggle for civilisation but is wheat our fine friend who has now outstayed its welcome in the 21st century?

Mankind became very adept at cultivating grains and progressively bred grains that were hardy and suited to particular climates (or continents). In the taxonomy diagram opposite you can see that wheat, barley and rye all share the same ancestral connections. So you can understand how all three are then jointly part of the problem of any subsequent diseases triggered by the consumption of grains (for example, coeliac disease).

Plant taxonomic classification, courtesy of Victor Zevallos

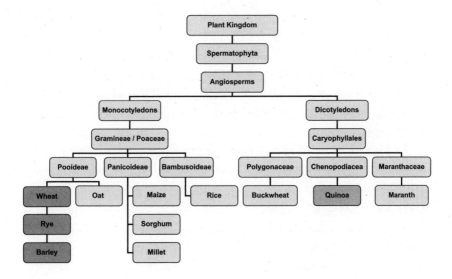

Contemporary trends in wheat production

Here is another historical fact that makes me wonder about whether our global consumption of wheat has increased. Prior to 1939 (and the outbreak of World War II) the rationing system had already been devised. This led to an imperative to try and increase agricultural production. Thus it was agreed in 1941 (in the UK) that there was a need to establish a Nutrition Society. A meeting of workers interested in nutritional problems was convened by Sir John Orr and was held at the Royal Institution.[12] The main objective of the new Society was to provide a common meeting place for workers in various fields of nutrition. The very roots of the Society were geared towards necessarily increasing the production of wheat. This goal was achieved and by the end of the 20th century, global wheat output had expanded five-fold.[13] Modern day global wheat production is considered to be over 700 million tonnes per year.[14] Now I should say that some quantity of this wheat would also be for animal feed and not just human consumption but there is no doubt that wheat has become a very significant staple part of our daily diets.

In Yuval Noah Harari's (Professor of History at the Hebrew University of Jerusalem) book *Sapiens: a brief history of humankind*, he makes an intriguing observation about wheat. He asserts that wheat had been insignificant in terms of its population of the earth but since the development of cultivation and agriculture it now covers 2.25 million square kilometres of the world. He asks the question that if wheat covers such a significant land mass and has humans in 'bondage' protecting it, ensuring it receives appropriate nourishment, nutrients and water, 'have these plants domesticated *Homo sapiens*, rather than vice versa?'

I hope I have convinced you that wheat has played such an influential role in the development and journey of humankind, and in the next section I would like to start to reveal the unforeseen consequences of this global expansion of wheat cultivation.

To understand 'gluten attack' we must first come to know coeliac disease

When and how did we first recognise coeliac disease?

Coeliac disease is considered to have first been described by Samuel Gee, a UK based physician from the 19th century. However, if we consider where the word 'coeliac' is derived from – coeliacus: new Latin from the Greek word koiliakos meaning abdominal – then we could suggest that our historical recognition of this condition dates back to the 1st or 2nd century AD. It was at this point that Aretaeus the Cappadocean described 'ventriculosa passio' (belly sickness) with features suggestive of malabsorption (malabsorption is a failure of our gut to absorb the nutrients which we consume). Samuel Gee acknowledged this early reference in his landmark lecture 'on the coeliac affection' which occurred at The Hospital for Sick Children, Great Ormond Street, London, on the

5th of October 1887. This report was subsequently published in the St Bartholomew's Hospital Reports.[15]

An extract from this report provides insight into the perception that coeliac disease was predominantly a paediatric condition and considered to only present with gastrointestinal manifestations and more specifically steatorrhoea (foul smelling stool which is linked to malabsorption). Here is an original extract from Gee:

> There is a kind of chronic indigestion which is met with persons of all ages, yet is especially apt to affect children between one and five years old. Signs of the disease are yielded by the faeces; being loose, not formed but not watery; more bulky than the food taken would seem to account for; pale in colour, as if devoid of bile; yeasty; frothy, an appearance probably due to fermentation; stinking, stench often very great, the food having undergone putrefaction rather than concoction … The onset is usually gradual, so that time is hard to fix: sometimes the complaint sets in suddenly, like an accidental diarrhoea; but even when this is so, the nature of the disease soon shows itself … The course of the disease is always slow, whatever be its end; whether the patient live or die, he lingers ill for months or years … But if the patient can be cured at all, it must be by means of diet.

Although Gee's description is historically accurate what is clear is that the coeliac disease we now see more than a century later is something quite different and far more diverse.

Willem Karel Dicke reported the next quantum leap, which occurred in our evolving knowledge of this condition.[16] Dicke was a general paediatrician working in Utrecht, Holland. His initial clinical observation was that there was considerable variation in the wellbeing of children at different times during their stay in hospital. Dicke correlated the mood alterations with variations in the stool weight and frequency. The diet of these children consisted of 'gruel'. This was a porridge-like substance which was common Dutch cuisine. Dicke enquired from the food preparation staff and discovered that the constituents of the 'gruel' varied depending on the availability of wheat flour. Legend would have it that this occurred in the 1940s when a constant supply of flour in Holland could not be guaranteed due to the Second World War. The story goes along the lines of Dicke observing an improvement in these children when there was no wheat available but when Americans dropped food parcels with wheat in, lo and behold the children's symptoms recurred. It is a nice story. The truth is that Dicke probably observed that children with significant gut symptoms when given gruel with a rice or potato flour base appeared to be far 'happier' than when eating the gruel based on wheat as far back as 1932, but like all medical research things take time to surface. Nevertheless, this unique clinical observation led to the recognition that a gluten-free diet was the cornerstone of management in coeliac disease.

However, it has been suggested that the effect of coeliac disease was present in the skeletal remains of a young lady from the 1st to the 2nd century AD. This archaeological report comes from Italy. [17] The site of the findings is a place historically known as Cosa on the Tyrrhenian coast near Tuscany. Cosa was founded in Roman times in 273 BC. The investigators uncovered a burial tomb that contained 37 skeletal remains. The diet of the time was predominantly a paleo diet (chiefly of meat, fish, vegetables and fruit, and excluding dairy or cereal products and processed food) although bread would have undoubtedly been available. In one of these skeletal remains a young woman had a very frail physique, short stature, thinning of bones, thin dental enamel and hip bone abnormalities. All of this could be consistent with malabsorption or chronic nutritional deficiencies. It is unlikely that this lady's appearance was due to starvation as she was buried in a richly decorated tomb with funeral artefacts considered by archaeologists to represent wealth. Furthermore other skeletal remains were not affected in the same way and this lady had the right genetic make-up for coeliac disease when her remains were tested accordingly. To provide isotope based scientific data the archaeologists looked at the presence of carbon and nitrogen in the bone samples. They found that this young lady's carbon content was low by comparison to her entombed co-residents while her nitrogen content was higher. These isotope findings can reflect markers of chronic malnutrition. For example, if you cannot absorb properly due to inflammation in your bowel this may lead to you breaking down skeletal muscle. Skeletal muscle is the largest reservoir for nitrogen that our body has, which in this lady's case results in a malnourished appearance while having a high isotope nitrogen level. Perhaps coeliac disease has been around for a very, very long time?

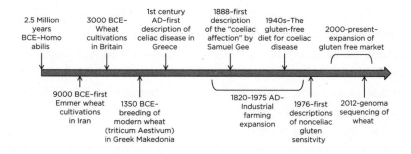

What is gluten?

There are so many answers for this with the obvious one being the 'devil'! ☺ Although I hope by now you have realised that this may not necessarily be the case and is not my view. I would simply like to give you the relevant scientific arguments and counter arguments which will allow you to decide. If you eat wheat then gluten is present

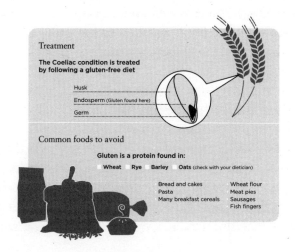

within this grain. A kernel of wheat contains the wheat husk, the embryo and the endosperm. Gluten is within the endosperm. The endosperm is the nutrient-rich tissue that surrounds the embryo and feeds the embryo. When considering the production of bread it is the endosperm that is ground down to make refined flour (see page 11).

The endosperm contains proteins which can be separated depending on their solubility in water or alcohol. From a biochemical perspective these high molecular weight proteins are alcohol soluble storage proteins and are called prolamins. The prolamins in wheat are called gliadins, for barley, hordeins, and for rye, secalins. All three have similar properties as they come from the same evolutionary production of grain (remember the left hand column from the taxonomy diagram on page 7). Why is this important? These prolamins contain gluten and through the industrial processing of wheat this is how gluten is separated from the rest of the grain so it can be used commercially.

From a food industry perspective gluten has excellent 'dough like' properties and this is viewed as highly desirable as it allows food manufacturers to make bread rise or give visco-elasticity to their food products. So it is not just bread that has gluten within it, many other products contain gluten often unbeknown to us. For example, breakfast cereals such as cornflakes, stock cubes, gravy granules, soya sauce, some ready meals, meat substitutes (the sort of stuff you will get in a takeaway pizza without realising it!), some energy drinks and my favourite, the Mars bar – incredible. So you start to get the picture of how liberally gluten is used within the food industry. Finally I would also mention that both medicines and cosmetics may contain gluten.

How do we develop coeliac disease?

So how does gluten cause coeliac disease? Step one for someone, anyone, to develop coeliac disease is that they need to have the right genetic profile. This genetic profile is described as HLADQ2 or DQ8 (Human Leucocyte Antigen). We all have HLA genes but there is a particular HLA code that associates itself with coeliac disease. Virtually everyone who has coeliac disease has this specific HLADQ2 or DQ8 gene code. My research group and others have historically shown that coeliac disease affects 1% of the population. Our work was a study undertaken between 1999 and 2001 but published in 2003 (it always takes a while to publish work in medical peer reviewed literature).[18] However, although 1% of the population have coeliac disease 25–40% of the population may have HLADQ2 or DQ8. So something else has to happen to these individuals beyond just having the right genetic appearance (let's call this the hidden step). I have termed it 'hidden' because none of the medical community is quite sure what the final trigger is. We know you have to have a certain genetic HLA code but we don't know why some develop coeliac disease and others don't.

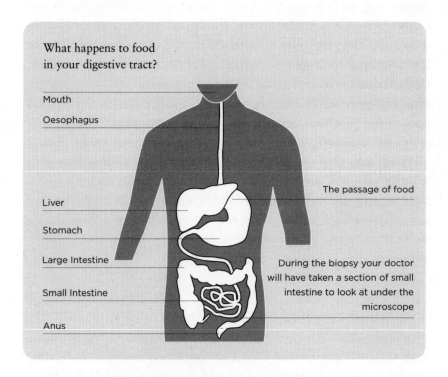

What happens to food in your digestive tract?

Mouth

Oesophagus

The passage of food

Liver

Stomach

Large Intestine

During the biopsy your doctor will have taken a section of small intestine to look at under the microscope

Small Intestine

Anus

Step two: an individual with HLADQ2 or DQ8 eats gluten and this is usually in the form of bread, pasta, pizza and so on. This food enters their stomach where the digestion process starts to take place. After the stomach the food will pass through the end of the stomach into the small bowel. Step three: the food is broken down into proteins called peptides which contain gluten. The small bowel is the hot house for the absorption of nutrients that are released through the digestive process. For us to maintain our nutritional status and not starve (in evolutionary terms) we need to absorb all the nutrients we can and for this reason the small bowel has evolved in a certain way. The small bowel is long – 3–5 metres – and has villi. Villi are microscopic finger-like structures that increase the surface area. I like to describe villi as seaweed floating or sea anemones in water grabbing things as they pass. After our food has passed through the digestive process and thus through the small bowel what is left enters the large bowel or colon. This is the part of the gastrointestinal tract which we investigate for colon cancer with national bowel cancer screening programmes. In the colon the 'waste' forms into stool or poo. The small bowel is approximately 3cm in diameter and the colon or large bowel is approximately 6cm in diameter, hence their historical medical names, but it is a source of amusement to me that the so called small bowel is the longest part of the gastrointestinal tract and has enough surface area to cover a tennis court! You can lose your entire colon and still stay alive but you cannot lose your small bowel. If you have less than 1 metre of small bowel for whatever reason then this is incompatible with life unless you are fed through an intravenous drip. I would not have called it the small bowel; I would have called it the larger than large bowel and blooming important!

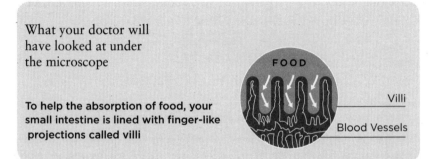

What your doctor will have looked at under the microscope

To help the absorption of food, your small intestine is lined with finger-like projections called villi

FOOD

Villi

Blood Vessels

Step four: these peptides cross the surface of the small bowel traversing the villi. The surface linings of the small bowel are called enterocytes and once the peptides have passed through this wall they are then presented to the HLADQ2 or DQ8. This results in the peptide or gluten stimulating our immune system. We have different immune cells circulating or living within our body – they are there to defend us and keep us well. You can imagine that as mankind was evolving we particularly needed a lot of these cells to be present in the gut. This would allow us to fight off infection. Gastrointestinal infections are likely to have been the biggest killer of evolving humankind and sadly are still a huge reason for death in poor income countries.

Step five: the particular immune cell which is critical to developing coeliac disease is called the T-cell. When presented with gluten the T-cell produces a whole immune response and stimulates attack cells that go back to the surface lining of the small bowel and destroy the villi. Step six: the attack cells within the lining of the small bowel are called intraepithelial lymphocytes or IELs. When these IELs go to work causing destruction in the small bowel we are left with an appearance which doctors call villous atrophy and I like to call flat bowel. Furthermore the unlucky person who develops coeliac disease also develops antibodies to gluten. We can test for these antibodies in your blood stream. There are many types which have been used over the years: gliadin antibodies, endomysial antibody, tissue transglutaminase antibodies and deamidated gliadin antibodies. So those are the six steps required to develop coeliac disease.[19] If you are a susceptible individual then the minute you eat gluten this cascade of events occurs in your body ultimately resulting in the development of coeliac disease. However bear in mind this only occurs in 1% of the population who actually develop coeliac disease. I hope I have made sense of this process and I have not confused you!

How does a doctor confirm the diagnosis of coeliac disease?

When a doctor wants to make a diagnosis of coeliac disease the first thing they do is to take a blood sample to look for one of the aforementioned antibodies. These antibodies do not clinch the diagnosis of coeliac disease but they point the way. However, it is critical that the doctor checks that the patient has not put him or herself on a gluten-free diet prior to the test. Now that I have described the immunological process and you know that the treatment for coeliac disease is the withdrawal of gluten, in other words a gluten-free diet, then I hope you will understand that if the blood sample is taken from someone who is on a self-imposed gluten-free diet, they may have a negative blood test even though they have undiagnosed coeliac disease!

So back to rule number one of Gluten Attack: if you have symptoms when you eat gluten don't place yourself on a gluten-free diet: please go and see a doctor.

If your family doctor or any other doctor you have seen has tested you for coeliac disease by doing a blood test and it is positive, then you require a camera test or gastroscopy in order to confirm the diagnosis. This is a fibre optic camera about 1cm in diameter and more than 1 metre in length which is initially placed into your mouth by a gastroenterologist (someone, like me, with a specialist interest in the gut). The gastroscopy may be performed with or without sedation depending on the patient's preference. The gastroscope is then passed from the mouth to just beyond the stomach entering the top end of the small bowel. The biopsies are taken from here. A biopsy is a small snip of tissue which we take from the small bowel. Each biopsy is usually about 2 millimetres in

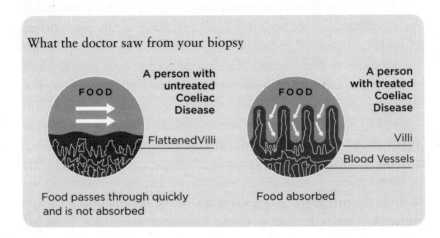

What the doctor saw from your biopsy

A person with untreated Coeliac Disease

FOOD

Flattened Villi

Food passes through quickly and is not absorbed

A person with treated Coeliac Disease

FOOD

Villi

Blood Vessels

Food absorbed

length. When we look at these biopsies under the microscope, instead of seeing lovely finger-like villi we see a flat bowel instead. A diagnosis of adult coeliac disease is therefore confirmed by having the combination of a positive antibody and a flat bowel on biopsy.

What are the symptoms of coeliac disease?

Individuals with coeliac disease can present to doctors in many different ways. Presenting with gut symptoms is common and an important point here is that the symptoms may be subtle. A few examples could be abdominal pain, bloating, diarrhoea, indigestion or irritable bowel type symptoms (IBS). However, even though the initial insult is to the gut, people with undiagnosed coeliac disease do not always have gut symptoms. For example, they may present with problems related to not absorbing nutrients, such as iron. The villi are flat and they have no means to pick up what their body needs by comparison to healthy individuals. Anaemia is a very common presenting feature of patients with coeliac disease. People who suffer with anaemia may not even know that they are affected but they may feel tired or complain of fatigue. Another feature of coeliac disease may be weight loss or failure to gain weight again due to the difficulties with absorption or malabsorption. If an individual is known to have coeliac disease then all their first-degree relatives, and by this I mean parents, brothers and sisters, and any children they may have, have a 10% risk of developing coeliac disease. Now this means they are at 10 times greater risk than the general population (because 1% of the population are affected), so this is another group of people for which doctors should have a low threshold for testing or if you like a higher degree of suspicion for coeliac disease.

Coeliac disease is an autoimmune disease: our own immune system turns on itself when we eat gluten. This means that other autoimmune diseases have an association with coeliac disease. For example, Type 1 diabetes, autoimmune thyroid disease, autoimmune hepatitis, primary biliary cirrhosis, rheumatoid arthritis, Sjogren's syndrome and systemic lupus erythematosus have all been linked to coeliac disease, although some of the associations are stronger than others. If we tested 100 patients with Type 1 diabetes for coeliac disease then 3–8 out of 100 may have coeliac disease. If you have one autoimmune disease you are more likely to have another by comparison to a person who has no history of autoimmune disease. I have always found it fascinating that unlike all the other autoimmune diseases you can shut coeliac disease down and recover by removing gluten from your diet. For every other autoimmune disease once you have started there is no stopping the process. You never stop having Type 1 diabetes. Your immune system continues to attack the pancreas (the organ which produces insulin) without hesitation.

Another fascinating but controversial observation is that investigators have suggested that having undiagnosed coeliac disease may promote the development of other autoimmune diseases in the affected individual. The researchers studied patients who have diagnosed coeliac disease and divided them into those who were diagnosed early (infancy) and those who were diagnosed in later life. The investigators reported that in their study of 909 coeliac patients the presence of other autoimmune diseases was 5.1% in those diagnosed under the age of 2 years, and 23.6% if you were older than 10 years at the time of diagnosis. The investigators put forward a theory that the longer you were exposed to gluten the more likely you were to develop other autoimmune diseases.[20] So it may be that gluten is opening the door through the gut and other autoimmune diseases follow.

To further this debate I want to tell you about a rare skin condition called dermatitis herpetiformis (DH). This is an itchy rash presenting with blisters typically on the buttocks, elbows, knees and sometimes your head. It was discovered that this skin condition had a unique relationship with coeliac disease. If you take a small bowel or duodenal biopsy from patients with DH then >70% will have the flat bowel of coeliac disease, but the other 30% will have the right genetics for coeliac disease (and perhaps the presence of the initial attack cells, the intraepithelial lymphocytes (IELs) I mentioned earlier) in the absence of villous atrophy. Thus it could be argued that all DH patients have coeliac disease or early coeliac disease. Furthermore this skin condition is treated by a combination of drugs and a gluten-free diet. So I consider the gut to be the point through which gluten 'breaks and enters'; thereafter how exactly different people present is not clear to me or indeed any other person researching in the field (beyond the six steps I outlined earlier), but it may be that it is about us as individual human beings. Perhaps different individuals – after going through the first six steps – then trigger different immune responses which determine whether you present with gut symptoms, anaemia, a skin rash or in another way.

What are the complications of coeliac disease and why should I go onto a gluten-free diet?

There are different aspects to consider when discussing a new diagnosis of coeliac disease with a patient. The first issue is complications. Patients will have often read on the internet that there is 'at least a two-fold increased risk of cancers or gut cancer'. This understandably freaks them out! However, a key point to make is the difference of *relative* risk and *absolute* risk. The statistic above suggests that if you have coeliac disease then by comparison to a person who does not have coeliac disease your risk of certain cancers is double or more. At face value for anyone that can be alarming. Now let's consider absolute risk. We all have a risk of cancer and it is a risk that increases with age. If I enter my details into an internet-based cancer risk calculator (from a reputable site) then my absolute risk of cancer is about 1 in 5,000. This means that for another person who is similar in every way to me (how unfortunate for them!), except that they have coeliac disease, then their absolute risk of cancer is twice that of mine. So their risk of cancer is 1 in 2,500. When you put it like that, as I do for patients when I counsel them in clinic, then it does not sound as terrifying. (By the way, if you are wondering and for the record, I don't have coeliac disease.)

So back to risk; there are other important and reassuring features which are essential to explain to our patients. It would appear that coeliac patients who are on a gluten-free diet and carefully adhere to it will reduce their risk of cancer with time, and that their risk becomes comparable to age- and sex-matched volunteers without coeliac disease. Essentially they switch off the inflammatory process by withdrawing gluten from their diet.

Another complication that may affect up to 40% of coeliac patients at the time of presentation is reduced bone mineral density. This is considered to be linked to malabsorption and the fact that with a flat bowel coeliac patients cannot necessarily absorb calcium as readily, leading to thinner bones. If your bones are a little thinner than they should be then this is called osteopenia; if it is more than this then it is called osteoporosis. Again this complication can be reduced, avoided or even reversed by commencing and adhering to a gluten-free diet. Other reasons to stick with the gluten-free diet are linked to the nutrient deficiencies I mentioned earlier and the fact that patients often feel tired if they have a shortage of iron, folate or vitamin B12.

When I discuss long-term complications with newly diagnosed coeliac patients I have noticed that for some of them this concept seems remote. Developing complications seems a long way away. This may not be the strongest reason for them to start a gluten-free diet. For me personally I would want to start a gluten-free diet to feel better. In other words, for the immediate improvement of my symptoms rather than the distant and perhaps theoretical benefit of avoiding complications. When I undertook my primary care study in 1999 trying to assess how common coeliac disease was I personally recruited 1,200 people.[18] I had some worries about this study as many of the people taking part said they felt completely well. I worried that I was taking healthy people and converting them into patients for the purpose of research. Twelve individuals were then found to have coeliac disease and commenced a gluten-free diet. I followed these patients up and the vast majority said that 'they felt better' on a gluten-free diet.[21] I was surprised by this given that so many at the start of the study said they felt completely well. How could this be? This is what the patients taught me: many said they had accepted their pre-coeliac diagnosis state as normal for them. From their perspective they 'did not know any better' and perhaps this was a level of wellbeing that they had come to accept as normal for them. The gluten-free diet was a revelation for many in terms of releasing new energy. A policeman who took part in this study said, 'I filled out the health questionnaire and said I was normal. Twelve months after the diagnosis of coeliac disease and being on the gluten-free diet I feel fantastic! I have a new lease of life. Previously I had accepted that I may need a nap after a busy day at work. We have two kids and at this middle age I thought that life is just busier, harder and more tiring. I gave up five-a-side football. Now I realise it was linked to coeliac disease. I feel amazing. I have gone back to playing football and have so much more energy. I wish I had been tested sooner.'

For me improving quality of life is the key. I would go onto a gluten-free diet in order to feel better, to gain energy, vitality and wellbeing.

If while reading this chapter you are thinking you have some of these problems or can relate to what is being described please go and see your doctor and ask if he/she would consider testing you for coeliac disease. I hope they would be receptive to the suggestion.

I'll end this section with one final fact. We have established that coeliac disease affects 1% of the adult population and there are numerous national and international guidelines that recommend testing for patients for coeliac disease who present with different symptoms. An example of this would be the National Institute of Clinical Excellence (NICE) Irritable Bowel Syndrome (IBS) guidelines published in 2008 and then again in 2015. The NICE guidelines explicitly state that patients with IBS type symptoms should be tested for coeliac disease (using the antibodies I mentioned before). However, at present in the UK only 1 in 5 individuals with coeliac disease have been diagnosed. There are likely to be between 400,000–500,000 people living in the UK alone who have not been diagnosed yet![22]

Rule number 3 of Gluten Attack:

It is okay for you to ask your doctor if you can be tested for coeliac disease.

The gluten explosion!

Changing trends in coeliac disease

Although I have mentioned that coeliac disease affects 1% of the population this was not the case historically. In 1950 the estimated incidence in the UK was reported as one in 8,000.[23] So what has happened in between?

Finland may serve to give us some clues. The population of Finland is a little over 5 million. The population is ethnically relatively homogenous. The country borders to the west with Scandinavian countries and to the east with Russia; the Finnish population is relatively stable with little migration. In 1980 the Finns undertook a screening study of coeliac disease and reported that their population prevalence was 1%; then more recently in 2000 they repeated their study and declared that the new prevalence of coeliac disease in Finland was 2%.[25] This represents a doubling in population prevalence over a 20-year period. The Finnish investigators also observed a very similar trend in the prevalence of Type 1 diabetes. In their report they present a clear figure of two parallel lines ascending over time representing the increase in prevalence for both coeliac disease and Type 1 diabetes. So their suggestion is that autoimmune diseases are on the rise and that both diseases they have studied reflect this. The theory behind this is that our immune systems are immunologically bored. As hunter gatherers the greatest threat to evolving mankind was that of gastrointestinal infection. Our immune system was geared up to fight infection, parasites and so on (as I said earlier). The small bowel is an entry point into our bodies and blood circulation, thus in order to protect us the small bowel is a very rich immunological area specifically to allow us to deal with the threat of infection. For argument's sake could I suggest to you that the Western world is an immunologically sterile environment? Perhaps our immune systems have nothing to do and are metaphorically twiddling their thumbs, because their challenges have all been historical? Infection is a thing of the past. In this environment is it possible that your immune system can turn on itself and you could develop an autoimmune disease? This theory has historically been known as the 'hygiene hypothesis' and was originally suggested by Professor David Strachan (Professor of Epidemiology at St George's, London, UK) in 1989.[26] Strachan made this suggestion with regards to allergic diseases but it was not long before this theory was extended to autoimmune diseases too. Strachan put forward the idea that we lost species diversity from the ecosystem of our own human body. Essentially the lack of early or childhood exposure to infectious agents and parasites stunts our human immune system's development. This means we cannot develop immune tolerance to these infectious agents (because for thousands of years this had been the main threat and we had biologically evolved to deal with this) and instead we have defects in our immune tolerance that open the door to allergy or autoimmune disease. You may have also heard of 'the biome depletion theory', or 'lost friends theory',[27] which are supportive views of the same story. This theory of 'hygiene hypothesis' is not without its critics. The idea that biome depletion or that loss of our human ecosystem occurred fitted with 20th century public health measures such as sewer systems and water treatment facilities, but in our modern society, hygiene has taken a more personal approach. Hand washing could be used as one example currently of great interest in hospital environments. Some scientists consider that 'modern hygiene' (such as hand washing) practices reduce exposure to allergens (like dust mite) and thus would have the opposite effect to increasing risk of allergy or autoimmune disease. They even raise concerns that the 'obsolete hygiene hypothesis' may have a negative effect on current public health measures and undermine modern public health strategy.

To push the debate forward with you I want to tell you about this study. A group of Australian-based researchers from Brisbane undertook a trial of giving patients with coeliac disease hookworm to see what effect it had on their underlying immune response. Hookworm of course is just the sort of parasite our forefathers had to deal with.[28]

This hookworm study was a randomised double blind placebo controlled trial. I want to break these components down for you as this is a recurring theme in scientific studies. Randomised means that participants agree to be randomly assigned to either arm of the study by chance; this is important to investigators. Investigators feel that this makes the study better, more scientific and more rigorous. For example, imagine I was going to ask a group of people which variety of cola drink they preferred by running a study in a local shopping mall. I am going to set up a stall and offer people passing by a drink of cola (Coke or Pepsi). Now just suppose I have worked out that people who come in the morning tend to be older while the late risers (after a fine night clubbing! ☺) tend to turn up in the afternoon. Furthermore imagine that I have heard the older population have a preference for Coke cola. So if I only conduct the study in the morning then my study may show that society has a preference for Coke cola. This would be a false result and not truly reflective of society. However, if I run the study all day and randomly allocate both cola varieties to participants this may show that both cola varieties are liked equally but that there is a preference revealed according to age. Without randomisation this would not have been observed.

So what does double blind mean? Double blind means neither the investigator nor the participant knows what they are receiving in the study. Back to the cola cans. To hide the identity of the cola would be important as we have suggested earlier that perhaps there may be a preference according to age. So now even if you start by saying you only like Coke cola, you don't know what you are drinking if it is presented to you in a Styrofoam cup. Blinding corrects our natural human bias. Equally the 'double' blind means I don't know which cola I am giving you. What if I really like Coke cola and keep saying to participants 'this is Coke cola, it's really lovely don't you think?' This would again influence the study and cause bias.

Finally let's discuss the placebo effect as this is a very important concept for science. Placebo in drug study terms is essentially something participants can be given which is inert or harmless. The reason for this is that participants can be influenced in a positive way by an intervention. For example, they may believe that by being given cola they feel much better, more alert because of the caffeine. So although participants report this, in fact I had actually given them blinded caffeine-free cola (as the placebo); this is the placebo effect.

We will return to my cola cans later on in this book –
I am really quite fond of them!

So back to the hookworm. A hookworm is a very common para-site globally (the fancy group name for this is Helminth), particularly in the developing world. Through its life cycle it lives in the soil and enters humans through the skin (you develop a rash). It can then migrate via our blood circulation to the small intestine where it attaches itself to the surface wall. This is where it has a preference to live and feed. If the environment is favoura-ble then it will release eggs passed out through our stool. Of course if this stool goes into the soil then the cycle can start all over again. The Brisbane investigators infected coeliac patients with hook-worm and then gave those coeliac patients a gluten challenge. In this small study they tried to demonstrate that the immunological response to gluten was less severe in the coeliac patients infected with hookworm by comparison to those given placebo. There was some signal in terms of both a reduced immunological response to the gluten challenge and less damage to the bowel when biopsies were taken. The Brisbane group is work in progress and judging by their publication stream they are still actively pursuing this theory, which of course supports the hygiene hypothesis. Coeliac patients with hookworm have got a bigger problem to deal with than those coeliac patients without hookworm who are just immunologically concentrating on themselves. This of course comes back to our theory of immune tolerance.

The effect of gluten in previously gluten-naïve cultures

There is another possibility to explain the increasing prevalence of coeliac disease and that is increasing gluten exposure. In 1999 a report was published in *The Lancet* suggesting that the endomysial antibody was present in 5.6% of the 989 children tested who lived in the Sahara Desert, and that the coeliac disease which had been suggested by antibody blood test was then confirmed by taking a small bowel biopsy.[29] The Saharawi tribe are an African population of the Western Sahara living in refugee camps due to political instability. Their staple diet in the refugee camp is wheat flour based. The investigators reported not only this high prevalence but also a very high HLA genetic predisposition by comparison to what I have previously described. The increased presence of the 'right' HLA (DQ2 or DQ8 if you recall earlier) in the Saharawi tribe is considered to be the result of consanguinity or intermarriage of familial members. So the increased prevalence of coeliac disease in the Saharawi tribe is likely to be due to a combination of both exposure to gluten and a population with a higher affinity for developing coeliac disease due to the HLA association.

Here is a similar story: Argentinian gastroenterology researchers have described their experience of an epidemic of coeliac disease in the Amerindian Toba community. These are impoverished indigenous people who have been hunter gatherers. With European colonisation they became dispossessed and attempted to live remotely. There are thought to be a little more than 60,000 surviving and they live in remote forest named locally as the 'Impenetrable'. Now in this modern era they have required governmental support. Since the government has provided them with nutritional support they have a completely different diet to their normal staple diet. The nutritional support that is given has been predominantly wheat based. The investigators have described astonishing gluten consumption per person as result of this government initiative. The average slice of bread is said to contain 2.5 to 3 grams of gluten, but for this population the consumption of gluten was 47 grams on average per day! Of the 143 people tested six had high antibodies for coeliac disease. This represents approximately 4% of the population tested. So in this small study (and I emphasise this so as not to overstate the observation) coeliac disease, a condition not previously reported, appears to be very common in these Amerindian indigenous people when given industrial quantities of gluten. This could be used to support a dose-dependent response to gluten which promotes the development of coeliac disease.[30]

Historically doctors from both China and the Indian sub-continent have virtually never reported coeliac disease as a significant problem. Very few cases have been described in the medical literature, until recently. Now we are seeing a fascinating development with progressive recognition of coeliac disease. What is happening? Here is my suggestion: both China and parts of the Indian subcontinent are changing their dietary habits; they have previously been predominantly rice based cultures. With globalisation has come global westernisation and I suggest that people from these cultures are now eating more bread, pizza and pasta. In other words, change to a wheat based culture and, voilà, coeliac disease follows.[31,32]

If we go all the way back in time to the 'Fertile Crescent' and how we got out of the hunter gatherer trap (page 6), you may recall that I suggested wheat was central to the process. Perhaps survival of the fittest occurred – if you had the right HLADQ2 or DQ8 for developing coeliac disease then this conferred a biological disadvantage to you. You were more likely to develop coeliac disease and, just like the young girl from Tuscany, your growth was stunted and you had nutritional deficiencies. You died young. The people with HLADQ2 or DQ8 genes were bred out or reduced in number within Western developing society. Now in present time when wheat is introduced to wheat-naïve cultures we see history repeating itself. Now I am not suggesting that changing your diet from rice to wheat is going to kill you in this modern world! However, it does appear to make you susceptible to developing coeliac disease.

There are alternative theories that are also worth discussing. One is the 'demic diffusion' by Cavalli-Sforza and Ammerman. This theory suggests that if the HLA prevalence of DQ2 and DQ8 was initially high in the Fertile Crescent and as these 'new' farmers expanded in numbers, they migrated into new lands that were relatively unpopulated and intermixed with other groups, all of which resulted in a progressive reduction in the HLADQ2 and DQ8 presence and thus a reduction in the occurrence of coeliac disease within these areas. Finally an intriguing observation about dental caries (or tooth decay) and HLADQ2 has recently been made. HLADQ2 may provide protection against dental caries.

Now dental caries in hunter gatherer humankind (evolving into farmers) is a really bad situation and could equate to starvation for those individuals affected. So historically the presence of HLADQ2 providing protection from dental caries may have conferred a survival benefit to those with HLADQ2 back in the mists of time. Irrespective of these theories one fact remains: if presented with enough gluten, where HLADQ2 (and DQ8) genes go, coeliac disease will follow.[33]

References

1. Sanders DS, Aziz I. Separating the wheat from the chat. *Am J Gastroenterol* 2012;**107**(12):1908-12.

2. http://www.trust.org/item/20150317194256-epmtq/?source= quickview

3. You Gov 2015.

4. Aziz I, Lewis NR, Hadjivassiliou M, Winfield SN, Rugg N, Kelsall A, Newrick L, Sanders DS. A United Kingdom study assessing the population prevalence of self-reported gluten sensitivity and referral characteristics to secondary care. *Eur J Gastroenterol Hepatol* 2014;**26**(1):33-9.

5. Burden M, Mooney PD, Blanshard R, White W, Cambray-Deakin D, Sanders DS. Cost and Availability of Gluten-free Food in the UK: In Store and Online. *Postgrad Med J* (*in-press July 2015*).

6. Cooper BT, Holmes GK, Ferguson R, Thompson R, Cooke WT. Proceedings: Chronic diarrhoea and gluten sensitivity. *Gut* 1976; **17**(5):398.

7. Ellis A, Linaker BD. Non-coeliac gluten sensitivity? *Lancet* 1978;**1**(8078):1358-9.

8. Cooper BT, Holmes GK, Ferguson R, Thompson RA, Allan RN, Cooke WT. Gluten-sensitive diarrhea without evidence of celiac disease. *Gastroenterology* 1980;**79**(5 Pt 1):801-6.

9. Falchuk ZM. Gluten-sensitive diarrhea without enteropathy: fact or fancy? *Gastroenterology* 1980;**79**(5 Pt 1):953-5.

10. Cooper BT, Holmes GK, Ferguson R, Thompson RA, Allan RN, Cooke WT. Gluten-sensitive diarrhea without evidence of celiac disease. *Gastroenterology* 1981;**81**(1):192-4.

11. Kaukinen K, Turjanmaa K, Mäki M, et al. Intolerance to cereals is not specific for coeliac disease. *Scand J Gastroenterol* 2000;35(9):942-6.

12. Copping AM. The history of the Nutrition Society. *Proc Nutr Soc* 1978;37:105-39.

13. International Maize and Wheat Improvement Center. *CIMMYT* 1998.

14. http://faostat.fao.org)

15. Gee S. On the coeliac affection. St Bartholomew's Hospital Reports; 1888; 24:17-20.

16. Dicke WK, Weijers HA, Van De Kamer JH. Coeliac Disease II; The presence in wheat of a factor having a deleterious effect in cases of coeliac disease. *Acta Paediatrica* 1953; 42:34-42.

17. Scorrano G, Brilli M, Martınez-Labarga C, Giustini F, Pacciani E, Chilleri F, Scaldaferri F, Gasbarrini A, Gasbarrini G, Rickards O. Palaeodiet Reconstruction in a Woman With Probable Celiac Disease: A Stable Isotope Analysis of Bone Remains From the Archaeological Site of Cosa (Italy). American Journal of Physical Anthropology 2015;154:349-56.

18. Sanders DS, Patel D, Stephenson TJ, Milford-Ward A, McCloskey EV, Hadjivassiliou M, Lobo AJ. A primary care cross-sectional study of undiagnosed adult coeliac disease. *Eur J Gastroenterol Hepatol* 2003;4:407-13.

19. Mooney PM, Hadjivassiliou M, Sanders DS. Coeliac Disease Clinical Review BMJ 2014 Mar 3;348:g1561. doi: 10.1136/bmj.g1561

20. Ventura A, Magazzu G, Greco L. Duration of exposure to gluten and risk for autoimmune disorders in patients with coeliac disease. Gastroenterology 1999;117:297-303.

21. Sanders DS, Hopper AD, Leeds JS, Hadjivassiliou M. Screening for coeliac disease – feasible and accurate but where does this novel technology take us? *BMJ* 2008;336:9.

22. West J, Fleming KM, Tata LJ, Card TR, Crooks CJ. Incidence and prevalence of celiac disease and dermatitis herpetiformis in the UK over two decades: population-based study. *Am J Gastroenterol* 2014;109: 757-68.

23. Davidson LSP, Fountain JR. Incidence of the sprue syndrome. *BMJ* 1950;1:1157-61.

24. Lohi S, Mustalahti K, Kaukinen K. Increasing prevalence of coeliac disease over time. *Aliment Pharmacol Ther*; 2007;26(9):1217-25.

25. Carpenter LI, Beral V, Strachan D, Ebi-Kryston KL, Inskip H. Respiratory symptoms as predictors of 27 year mortality in a representative sample of British adults. *BMJ* 1989;299(6695):357-61.

26. Rook GA, Martinelli R, Brunet LR. Innate immune responses to mycobacteria and the down regulation of atopic response. *Curr Opinion Allergy Clin Immunol* 2003;3:337-442.

27. Daveson AJ, Jones DM, Gaze S, McSorley H, Clouston A, Pascoe A, Cooke S, Speare R, Macdonald GA, Anderson R, McCarthy JS, Loukas A, Croese J. Effect of hookworm infection on wheat challenge in celiac disease – a randomised double-blind placebo controlled trial. *PLoS One*. 2011: 8;6(3):e17366. doi: 10.1371/journal.pone.0017366.

28. Croese J, Giacomin P, Navarro S, Clouston A, McCann L, Dougall A, Ferreira I, Susianto A, O'Rourke P, Howlett M, McCarthy J, Engwerda C, Jones D, Loukas A. Experimental hookworm infection and gluten microchallenge promote tolerance in celiac disease. *J Allergy Clin Immunol* 2015;135:508-16.

29. Catassi C, Rätsch IM, Gandolfi L, Pratesi R, Fabiani E, El Asmar R, Frijia M, Bearzi I, Vizzoni L. Why is coeliac disease endemic in the people of the Sahara? *Lancet* 1999:21;354(9179):647-

30. Va Quez H, Temprano M de L, Sugai E, Scacchi SM, Souza C, Cisterna D, Smecuol E, Moreno ML, Longarini G, Mazure RM, Bartellini MA, Verdú EF, González A, Mauriño EC, Bai JC. Prevalence of celiac disease and celiac autoimmunity in the Toba native Amerindian community of Argentina. *Can J Gastroenterol* July 2015 (E-pub ahead of print).

31. Wang XQ, Liu W, Xu CD, Mei H, Gao Y, Peng HM, et al. Celiac disease in children with diarrhea in 4 cities in China. *Journal of Pediatric Gastroenterology and Nutrition* 2011;53(4):368-70.

32. Kochhar R, Sachdev S, Kochhar R, Aggarwal A, Sharma V, Prasad KK, et al. Prevalence of coeliac disease in healthy blood donors: a study from north India. *Dig Liv Dis* 2012;44(6):530-2.

33. Catassi C, Gatti S, Lionetti E. Co-localization of gluten consumption and HLA-DQ2 and -DQ8 genotypes, a clue to the history of celiac disease. *Dig Liver Dis* 2014;46(12):1057-63.

CHAPTER 2

Breaking bread

The title I always wanted for the book but was wisely guided away!

Bread is central to mankind's existence. It has transcended its role as a food. Let me give you an example: 'We broke bread together.' This is an expression which denotes friendship or a closeness of relationship by the act of eating together. Central to the Christian religion and indeed other religions is the sharing of bread as an act of faith. 'When He had taken some bread and given thanks, He broke it and gave it to them, saying, this is my body which is given for you; do this in remembrance of me.' This is taken from the Bible, New Testament, Luke chapter 22 verse 19. This is the central act of communion. There are even colloquial expressions that use bread as a metaphor: 'Have you got any dough?' Once again this reveals how bread is of such importance to society that it has become a slang substitute for money. Why are there so many different ways to talk about bread in different aspects of our culture? Perhaps the historical concept of 'Bread and Circuses' best denotes the significance of bread to our society. It is something which I learnt from a dear friend. Bread and Circuses derives its meaning from Ancient Rome. It is a form of political distraction or appeasement. Juvenal (*circa* AD 100) was a Roman satirical poet and he suggests that the common Roman citizens can be appeased during times of peace by providing food (bread) and entertainment (circuses). This acts as a distraction from more significant political and societal issues which may be happening right under their noses. Strikes me society and politics has not changed over the millennia! Why was it bread that was given to the public? It is because starvation or hunger was a reality of ancient times and bread was one of the most available mass produced foodstuffs even in Ancient Rome. Bread was if you like a currency for survival all unto itself. Finally perhaps my favourite example of this was 'Let them eat cake' (okay I am cheating as it is not strictly bread!), allegedly attributed to Queen Marie Antoinette as an act of disregard towards the famine ridden peasants during the time of the French Revolution. On my research journey I realised there was little evidence to support the assertion that it was indeed Marie Antoinette's comment but nevertheless this comment is still considered to have historical symbolic importance. Pro-revolutionary historians cite this quote as the evidence for selfishness of the French upper classes at that time who could eat cake (or brioche) while the common people of French society were suffering. It is considered during that time that 'the staple food of the French peasantry and the working class was bread, accounting for 50 percent of their income, as opposed to 5 percent on fuel; the whole topic of bread was therefore of obsessional national interest' (*Marie Antoinette: The Journey* by Antonia Fraser, Orion publishing group). To this day we use this expression of 'let them eat cake'.

What all of this signifies is the historical, cultural and political significance of bread. Yet we now see a strong movement towards suspicion of bread and of course other gluten containing foods. This is wonderfully depicted in a recent website which provides humorous images of great art with all traces of gluten removed: http://glutenimage.tumblr.com/

So what has happened in between?

Ancient grains

The original Einkorn wheat (*Triticum baeoticum*, or its domesti-cated form, *Triticum monococcum*) is virtually never produced commercially. Einkorn wheat is considered one of the first plants to be domesticated and farmed in the Fertile Crescent. Einkorn is a short plant about 70cm or a little more than 2 feet high and produces a limited number of edible seeds. Emmer wheat is another similar original plant of the Fertile Crescent (domesticated species are *Triticum turgidum* subsp. *dicoccum* and *Triticum turgidum conv. Durum* and the wild species is called *Triticum turgidum* subsp. *Dicoccoides*). The first step of domestication of these wheat plants was to breed a variety of Einkorn or Emmer which did not shed its seeds spontaneously; by achieving this our ancient farming ancestors could ensure controlled harvesting and maximise the amount of grain which they collected. Thereafter we became more and more ingenious at selective breeding, hybridisation, cross fertilisation and many other techniques which maximised our yield of wheat (see page 7).

There is a suggestion that our modern cultivation practices have led to wheat which has an enriched gluten content. Dr William Davis termed this 'Frankenwheat' in his book *Wheat Belly* 2011. This is difficult for me to clarify despite looking extensively at the scientific literature. There is no doubt that the appearance of modern wheat may be short and stocky and that it may have a high grain yield; however, I am unable to clarify if there is increased gluten content. I am afraid there is no published literature to support this assertion. A recent publication from Professor Chibbar (University of Saskatchewan, Canada) is enlightening. Chibbar's group looked at the protein content of different varieties of wheat planted in North America since the 19th century. They hypothesised that if the gluten content has increased in wheat then by using biochemical techniques they would be able to demonstrate increased levels of protein in the more contemporary varieties (because gluten is a protein).[1] What they found was that protein levels in wheat increased by about 0.01% per year. This is incredibly low. So the issue of Frankenwheat remains controversial but I like the term!

Another alternative which is both supported and refuted within the scientific community is that ancient grains are not as toxic as the modern varieties. This is based on studies looking at the immunological response of patients with coeliac disease who are exposed to both modern and ancient grains. I think it would be fair to say that the jury is still out on this particular scientific perspective.

Bread making processes

The role of gluten may have changed when considering the industrial manufacturing of bread. Bread making involved the addition of yeast to make the bread ferment and thereafter rise. This is what separated unleavened bread from the bread we commonly eat. Of course bread rising requires gluten because of its dough-like viscoelastic properties.

In the UK in 1961 the British Baking Industries Research Association (based at Chorleywood, Hertfordshire, UK) created the 'Chorleywood process': this process allowed the rapid fermentation of bread which takes a matter of hours and as you can imagine this has huge economic advantages in comparison to traditional bread making. This rapid process is achieved by mechanical high speed mixers but also the suggestion of higher gluten content to enhance viscosity. This is not *The Great British Bake Off* or indeed any other television programme across the globe where dough is lovingly kneaded!

The average amount of gluten in a slice of bread is historically said to be 2.5 to 3 grams. However, if you go into any supermarket today and look at the selection of breads available and then study gluten content it is simply not reported. Calorie content, fibre, quantity of fat or salt is all listed, but not gluten. So this may equate to increased gluten consumption through the modern industrial bread making process without us even knowing.

Further evidence to support this could come from observations about sourdough bread. Sourdough is made with naturally occurring lactobacilli and yeast, and this process takes time but some may say it enhances taste. Italian investigators demonstrated that a 60-day diet of baked goods made from hydrolyzed wheat flour with sourdough lactobacilli and fungal protease did not cause immunological toxicity to patients with coeliac disease.[2]

Germany is viewed as a significant consumer of sourdough and Germany is also reported to have low rates of coeliac disease compared to the rest of Europe. So the interesting suggestion here is that our contemporary industrial bread making process requires more gluten and this in turn could be responsible for the shift or increased presence of both coeliac disease and perhaps other gluten related problems.

You, insects and gluten

Why does wheat have gluten? Previously I have mentioned that gluten is within the endosperm of the wheat grain and acts as a storage protein to feed the embryo (see page 11). This is one reason biologically why gluten exists, but another is protection. Gluten is indigestible for most insects although there are a few such as the *Nysius huttoni* (wheat bug) or *Eurygaster integriceps* (sunn pest or corn bug) who can eat wheat. The presence of indigestible gluten within the wheat grain provides protection from insects and confers a biological advantage to wheat and other gluten-containing grains. Humans are also unable to digest gluten but this did not stop us eating wheat! We can break down other proteins to their basic building blocks that are called amino acids but we cannot do this with gluten: it reaches a certain protein configuration of many protein blocks and will not allow itself to be digested further. In fact it is this aspect of gluten which is the problem or 'antigen' (something foreign to be attacked) to our immune system.

So it is not clear to me whether there are varieties of wheat that are more gluten enriched, or if our bread making *process* is the culprit. What is clear to me is that since we first isolated gluten in 1745 we understood its nature and value.[3] We have exploited its properties ever since and it may simply be that we are eating industrial quantities of gluten. Unbeknown to us, gluten is ubiquitous. It is considered that we eat 15 to 20 grams per day and this may not all be in bread.[4] Vital gluten (as it is sometimes called) is used in the food industry for sauces, instant soups and even medication. This may be central to the issue of Gluten Attack and account for a significant amount of our unwitting gluten consumption.

References

1. Hucl P, Briggs C, Graf RJ, Chibbar RN. Genetic gains in agronomic and selected end-use quality traits over a century of plant breeding of Canada Western Red Spring Wheat. Cereal Chemistry Accepted for Publication 2015 http://dx.doi.org/10.1094/CCHEM-02-15-0029-R.
2. Greco L, Gobbetti M, Auricchio R, Di Mase R, Landolfo F, Paparo F, Di Cagno R, De Angelis M, Rizzello CG, Cassone A, Terrone G, Timpone L, D'Aniello M, Maglio M, Troncone R, Auricchio S. Safety for patients with celiac disease of baked goods made of wheat flour hydrolyzed during food processing. *Clin Gastroenterol Hepatol* 2011;9(1):24-9.
3. Beccari B. De frumento. In: De Bononiensi Scientiarum et Artium Instituto atque Academia Commentarii: Bononiae: ex typographia Laelii a Vulpe; 1745.
4. Tjon JM, van Bergen J, Koning F. Celiac disease: how complicated can it get? *Immunogenetics* 2010;62(10):641-51.

CHAPTER 3

Sizing up gluten sensitivity

The dilemma of Djokovic

As a doctor I have been seeing patients with coeliac disease or suspected coeliac disease for more than 20 years. Many patients have come to me during this time saying they had symptoms related to eating gluten. I understood that to make a diagnosis of coeliac disease you needed a positive blood test and a biopsy of your small bowel taken with an endoscope. This is conventional medical practice the world over. It is essential to get the diagnosis correct at the outset. Why? So medical doctors like myself can give the appropriate advice about complications, risk of coeliac disease to other members of the family, long-term benefits of a gluten-free diet – all the things I mentioned earlier. I labour the importance of a cast iron diagnosis because of these issues. Recently I have read the account of Novak Djokovic having the diagnosis of coeliac disease suggested to him on the basis of applied kinesiology. Applied kinesiology is an alternative medicine technique that suggests illness or selects treatments for an individual patient based on the strength or weakness of muscle testing. So how did this apply to Djokovic? His account is very clear; he felt strongly that his playing level was not reaching its maximum capacity despite his best efforts. In July 2010 at a tournament in Croatia, Djokovic's doctor (Dr Cetojevic) asked him to place his left hand on his stomach and raise his right hand. Dr Cetojevic asked Djokovic to stop him pushing his right arm down. Having established that Djokovic could oppose the pushing down of his right arm, Dr Cetojevic then asked Djokovic to place a slice of bread against his stomach. This time Djokovic noticed a fundamental difference in terms of strength in his right arm muscles. Thus the sensitivity to gluten was discovered. Djokovic grew up in Serbia, a country where bread is an important staple and a daily part of the Serbian diet. So in that moment, from Djokovic's perspective, he started on a journey of recognition of the previously hidden barrier to his peak performance, which has ultimately led to his unparalleled tennis success. Novak Djokovic did go on to have blood testing for gluten related antibodies but I have read his book carefully and searched other sources (whether newspapers or internet), and I am as yet unable to find any evidence that he ever had a gastroscopy and biopsy. So we cannot tell whether Novak Djokovic has coeliac disease or gluten sensitivity. My guess is we will never know and the rest, as they say, is history.

I think it is worth clarifying my opinions of complementary and alternative medicine at this stage. I have no negative views whatsoever and in fact think these may provide excellent additional therapies for a variety of conditions. The critical point in this instance for me is that the diagnosis of coeliac disease does not appear to have been excluded. If this has not occurred then there is the risk that Western medical practice clashes with complementary and alternative medicine. I hope you as the reader agree with me and think my view is both a reasonable perspective and pragmatic?

The first steps towards recognising gluten sensitivity?

I had noticed in my own practice that patients were attending appointments having self-reported or self-diagnosed symptoms when they eat gluten. In hindsight and to my shame I suspect I did not take this as seriously as I should have, unless I made a diagnosis of coeliac disease in such patients. For the rest I would simply explain to them that they did not have coeliac disease. At that time this was within the bounds of conventional medicine (and my wisdom or imagination)!

Growing up, my amazing father – a distinguished physician – had quite a job rearing me (more shame on my part I am afraid). I think it would be fair to say that I was errant and let's leave it at that. On one occasion I told him that I had little belief or respect for wisdom: 'a stupid young man just becomes a stupid old man' I said. 'Really?' my father said looking at me questioningly. 'Well then, son, that leaves no hope for you,' he declared with a wide smile on his face. I now understand that wisdom is accumulated experience, and finally the penny has dropped with gluten sensitivity. I started to step away from what I was taught didactically during my medical training and instead asked open questions about what I was seeing and hearing from patients. Over a seven-year period I collected all the patients I had seen who presented having self-reported symptoms related to the consumption of gluten. I then undertook a population survey of the general public to assess the prevalence of self-reported symptoms when eating gluten. We published our work and there were three key messages. First, the public were (and still are) self-reporting symptoms to gluten at a high level, 13% in our UK survey published in 2014. Secondly, 2.9% of the general public are on a gluten-free diet even though they do not have coeliac disease. Thirdly, the demographics of the secondary care patients (in other words patients who have been referred by their general practitioner to the hospital for a specialist opinion) who presented with gluten sensitivity were very similar to the people who were describing symptoms in the population survey. This is important as it lends strength to our observations. It is a form of triangulation if you wish. I would like to talk about the secondary care patients and describe them a little. In these 200 patients the sex ratio was predominantly female, average age 30s to 40s and a high prevalence of irritable bowel type symptoms. We compared this group to patients I diagnosed with coeliac disease during the same time frame. The first thing we noticed which was encouraging if you have gluten sensitivity was that these patients did not commonly have the nutritional and metabolic deficiencies of patients with coeliac disease. The gluten sensitivity patients generally did not have anaemia, their iron stores were usually not low and they did not usually have low vitamin B12 levels. This was important clinical information and I think reassuring to patients with gluten sensitivity. Another important feature of these patients was that almost 50% of the gluten sensitivity patients had the genetic association with HLADQ2 or DQ8 that is necessary to develop coeliac disease. So as a preliminary observation it could be suggested that there is some demographic and genetic overlap between patients with coeliac disease and those with gluten sensitivity. This was the first categorisation of such adult patients to be reported in tandem with population prevalence.

The way this affected my practice was that I would of course still exclude coeliac disease (if right to do so) in patients who reported symptoms when eating gluten, but once I had done this I would advise patients that they had gluten sensitivity. I would explain that this was an area that we were only starting to understand. I would explain that currently this was a diagnosis of exclusion as we had no specific test that we could use to recognise gluten sensitivity. I would reassure them that the data we had published suggested that the consequences and complications that are reported in patients with coeliac disease do not occur with the same frequency in gluten sensitivity. Furthermore this meant they did not necessarily have to adhere to a gluten-free diet with the same degree of rigidity as recommended for coeliac patients; it could even mean that in the future their sensitivity may change and lifelong adherence may not be necessary. Ultimately I would encourage the patients to work with the diagnosis and adhere at a level that suited them and improved their symptoms. Although I am not sure we appreciated this at the time, in many ways it was a landmark study.

The *British Medical Journal* (*BMJ*) is a journal I have a remarkable fondness and liking for. I am sure this is a sentimental reason as it is the journal you first get when you become a doctor in the UK and join the British Medical Association (BMA). The *BMJ* drops through the post box of almost 120,000 doctors and is read by far more via the internet and overseas. I also like it because it is, in my opinion, unique. A few years ago the previous editor of the *BMJ* came under fire for changing the format of how research was presented. Instead of full papers with every detail (which is conventional) they opted for broadly a one-page summary. This was viewed as 'dumbing down' by many in the medical community. Doctor Richard Smith, the editor of the time, said something like this in response to the criticism (I am paraphrasing here based on my memory): 'the *BMJ* is a high impact credible scientific medical journal, the *BMJ* is a magazine, the *BMJ* is a rag. The *BMJ* provides information to primary care, to secondary care and to researchers. The *BMJ* is today's hot news and tomorrow's chip paper [in the UK we have a tradition of using newspaper to serve fish and chips]. The *BMJ* is all things to all men.' A colleague of mine had once said to me 'if you publish in *The Lancet* you will become a Professor but if you publish in the *BMJ* you will be famous'.

On the back of the prevalence study (which I first mentioned in Chapter 1, reference 4) we were asked to write an article entitled 'Does gluten sensitivity exist in the absence of coeliac disease?' The *BMJ* are brilliant at controversy and gave this article an associated front cover, a picture of a slice of bread with the words written across 'The challenge of non-coeliac gluten sensitivity'. It topped the most frequently read article for the *BMJ* for quite some time, which I think reflects both interest and controversy.[1,2]

References

1. Aziz I, Hadjivassiliou M, Sanders DS. Uncertainties page: Does non-coeliac gluten sensitivity exist? *BMJ* 2012;345:e7907. doi: 10.1136/bmj.e7907.
2. Spence D. Bad Medicine: Food Intolerance. *BMJ* 2013;346:f529 doi: 10.1136/bmj.f529.

CHAPTER 4

Do you have food intolerance, are you wheat allergic or is this a lifestyle choice?

Bad press

The confusion surrounding gluten sensitivity is a double-edged sword. In 2004 we historically reported that UK chefs had less knowledge than the general public with regards to coeliac disease. The lower the price ticket of your meal, the greater the risk of being told there was no gluten, before then being glutened! Patients have repeatedly described this to me and coined the phrase of being 'glutened', so I decided to study this formally. If there were a food equivalent of Russian roulette then for people with coeliac disease this would be carry out food or takeaway food! So great was their concern that this actually restricted coeliac patients' dietary habits and social life.[1] They were less likely to eat out or even go round to a friend's house than individuals who did not have coeliac disease. The increasing rise of interest in and recognition of gluten sensitivity has greatly improved this situation. Market forces have responded to gluten sensitivity by providing more choice and the knowledge base of chefs and the public alike has greatly increased over the ten years since our initial report.[2] Now here is the down side or kick back: there is a belief that many individuals who go gluten-free are on the latest food fad, the current 'in diet', celebrity endorsed and market driven band wagon. What evidence do we have to this effect? Firstly the increasing consumer trends for a gluten-free diet which I reported in Chapter 1. Secondly, what little data there is suggests that there are other reasons than just medical symptoms which make us choose to try a gluten-free diet, for example the perception that this may allow us to reduce our calorie intake, weight watching or the belief that 'free from anything is just simply healthier'.[3] We anecdotally reported, in a New York restaurant a coeliac patient, when asking for a gluten-free menu, was questioned by the waitress 'is that health or lifestyle?'[4] This perhaps summarises either the possible discrimination or judgement patients may face as well as the clinical conundrum that clinicians have a duty to clarify for society as a whole.

What is food allergy?

So this brings me to terminology. One-fifth of the population are considered to have adverse reactions to food. A reaction to food is nothing more than a generic term and needs to be qualified as there are different types of 'reactions'. Let's start with food allergy, which is a very specific term. Food allergy is an immunological response to a particular food substance and can be diagnosed by the presence of a particular antibody: the IgE antibody (completely unrelated to the antibodies seen in coeliac disease). The IgE antibody is produced in response to an antigen (a foreign substance to be attacked which was something I mentioned earlier on page 35). It is part of our immune protection system and there are different types, IgE being one type. It is really important for me to clarify this issue of IgE antibody. You can be tested for food allergy formally through your family doctor (general practitioner in the UK). You will be referred to the local immunology unit which will be in a secondary care setting, in other words a hospital. The tests for IgE mediated food allergy are the skin prick test or measuring in your blood stream (serology) food-specific IgE antibody levels. Now here is a really, really important diagnostic point. The main difficulty with both skin prick tests and IgE serological testing is that you can be sensitised to a food allergen but not have a food allergy. What do I mean by this? Many of us will have positive IgE antibodies or prick test if we are tested but may not have any symptoms whatsoever. We have been sensitised at some point in our immunological history but have not developed an allergy. So it is essential to be seen by an expert to make the diagnosis of food allergy. This diagnosis is made by the combination of the patient's history of an allergic response following the ingestion of specific foods and the positive IgE test. Typical symptoms and signs related to food allergy are tingling or itching in the mouth, hives (urticaria), itching or eczema, swelling of the lips, face, tongue and throat or other parts of the body (angioedema), wheezing, nasal congestion and of course gastrointestinal symptoms such as abdominal pain, diarrhoea, nausea or vomiting. Other supportive aspects of the history for patients with food allergy may be the presence in that individual or their family of atopic conditions such as asthma, hay fever, eczema or allergic rhinitis. Given this diversity of symptoms and the fact that individuals can be sensitised without having allergy you can then see how the diagnosis may not be as straightforward as we may think. This is why the double blind placebo controlled food challenge is viewed as the gold standard by doctors. What makes testing even harder is that this gold standard has a risk of anaphylaxis.[5] Anaphylaxis is an extreme form of hypersensitivity: the IgE antibody is in overdrive and switches on a particular cell called a mast cell. You will have heard of mast cells with regard to hay fever. So the mast cells contain histamine and it releases histamine in industrial quantities. Anaphylaxis has the rare risk of cardiorespiratory collapse or cardiac arrest.

IgE mediated food allergy is classically described in infants or children. IgE food allergy is said to affect 4–7% of preschool kids. Common examples which you would be familiar with are cow's milk allergy, peanut, other forms of nuts from trees (cashews, brazils, pistachio and pecan are some examples), egg, shellfish and some forms of tinned fish. Food allergy appears to be far less common in adults, perhaps 1–2%. The reasoning behind this comes back to what I had said earlier, on page 23, about 'immune tolerance'. Immune exposure to food is part of our normal biological process and starts after birth when we start to eat. Our immune system recognises the dietary proteins present in what we eat and under normal circumstances will in due course develop immune tolerance and accept the foods we are eating without developing the allergic reactions I described earlier. This process takes time, hence food allergy diminishes when progressing into adult life as our immune tolerance increases.[6]

Oral allergy syndrome and food dependent exercise-induced anaphylaxis

We are all familiar with hay fever, asthma and allergic rhinitis, whether as sufferers or not. The concept of seasonality to these conditions is also both recognised and accepted. Here is an interesting condition I came across while undertaking research for this chapter. Oral allergy syndrome is sometimes also called pollen food allergy. Pollen sensitised individuals may develop symptoms when they eat certain fruit and vegetables. The reason for this is that their immune system which is already IgE charged against pollen falsely recognises some fruit and vegetables in a similar way, again mounting an IgE response. The symptoms are thought to be more prolific or severe when the pollen count is high in much the same as hay fever.

These unfortunate individuals describe symptoms of an allergic phenomenon affecting their lips, mouth and throat. Those affected typically describe allergic type symptoms of itching and tingling. Once again there is the rare possibility of anaphylaxis. Oral allergy syndrome is considered to affect up to 2% of the UK population and has an association with birch tree pollen. Individuals who have birch pollen allergy are said to have oral allergy syndrome in 50% to 90% of cases.

Food dependent exercise-induced anaphylaxis is a rare disorder affecting both children and adults. The presentation by patients is quite amazing: they give a very specific description of allergic symptoms which occur during or after exercise. The symptoms are as I described for anaphylaxis earlier in this chapter involving skin, breathing and gastrointestinal symptoms. For these individuals there is a history of eating the offending food, typically two hours prior to exercise but this may even occur if they eat the food allergen after exercise. Standard food allergy testing is appropriate and the usual suspected food allergens are listed such as shellfish, peanuts and such like. Wheat is also very commonly linked under these circumstances and this is something I would like to come back to shortly.

On my soap box

I hope you will allow me a brief but for me important word about testing for these conditions. In the UK I see patients not infrequently who say they have had X test performed which suggested symptoms related to Y food or substance. They may even provide me with a detailed printout of their analysed samples which they were sent through the post or had taken via a private consultation. I always feel very sad when this happens and I don't mean this in a patronising way. For me this suggests that our conventional medical approach has failed and, particularly in the UK where the National Health Service (NHS) is free at the point of contact, this suggests desperation from that person's perspective. They want to find out what the problem is and they want to feel better. If the medical system is not helping them then they are trying to help themselves. You cannot chastise anyone for that but the problem is that we come back to the 'Cold War' of conventional Western medical practice versus complementary and alternative medicine. The patient crosses this boundary by using an unconventional test or consulting with a complementary or alternative practitioner and unwittingly falls foul of the system. The patient has entered 'No man's land', a place where your consultation with the enemy (by this I mean an alternative medicine practitioner) has made your attempt to re-enter the conventional medical system null and void. Once again I restate my position on this as per the previous chapter (just in case you have flicked the book open to this chapter and are already feeling your temperature rising when you read this paragraph!). I have no negative views whatsoever of complementary and alternative medicine and in fact think these may be excellent additional therapies for a variety of conditions. The critical point here for me is that the correct diagnosis of X has been made. If it has not then there is a risk that the patient may be given the wrong diagnosis and at that point Western medical practice clashes with alternative medicine.

The concern is this: many of the tests available through the internet lack any validation process. What do I mean by this? If you have a new medical test the first thing you do is compare it against the established gold standard. If it compares favourably, for example it is just as good at detecting the condition you are looking for, then this is encouraging. Your next step is to publish your work in the medical literature. This means your work undergoes a peer review by experts who will scrutinise the data. This process is very good for patients in my opinion. It comes back to the vow I and my colleagues took at medical school graduation *'Primum non nocere'*: first do no harm. Following peer review if your work is accepted for publication in a journal then it is accessible on an internet medical search engine which every doctor uses: PubMed or *medline*.

Now we have to be careful about this process of scientific validation. Industry has latched onto this concept and they can be crafty. I recently watched an advert for a brand of yoghurt with 'good bacteria' in it. The advert was sharp, it had style, there were attractive people like you and me (actually much, much, much better looking and better dressed than I will ever be!) expounding the benefits of having taken this product. They looked so happy, so well, the marketing men and women had done their job to an exemplary standard. These 'ordinary' people looked great and therefore just by having this yoghurt I too could look great. All I have to do is take one simple step – go out and buy this yoghurt at once. If I go out and buy this product immediately, I will feel better, look better, people may actually like me and I may even dress better! ☺ The headline on the advert was something like this, 'more than 70% of people tested said this yoghurt improved their gut symptoms'.

However, in small print at the bottom of the screen it said the number tested was something like 96! Furthermore, when you looked at the choices available to participating individuals when asked the question about improving their gut symptoms, they were given three choices; definite improvement, some improvement and no improvement. So there is a two out of three chance of the answer for the company being 'improved gut symptoms'. This is what is called in my business a positive ascertainment bias. It gives a high chance of getting the answer you wanted. Why don't you try this at home? Serve your friend or partner something they are not that fond of eating and then ask them 'did you think that was a nice meal I made?' Two out of three times or more they will say 'yes', or 'it was quite good'; you have made it hard for them to say no. An open question like 'what did you think of the meal?' does not have a positive ascertainment bias. So let's come back to the yoghurt. Could the UK public change its habits based on this level of data? Maybe yes, we will, if it is presented to us in what I would describe as a slightly disingenuous way. Media and marketing is powerful and can override the facts or truth. This is human nature I believe and we don't need to look deeply at medicine for this: just look across at the world of politics every day. What if I told you that there is scientifically validated and published data revealing that the vast majority of 'live bacteria' in yoghurts are killed by acid produced by the stomach after you have eaten it? What if I told you that by marketing these products under the banner of food supplement rather than drug it allows manufacturers to evade the normal stringent assessments made for any new drug? Would you be amazed by these two facts which have completely failed to penetrate general society while live bacteria yoghurts have proliferated within popular culture and have been accepted by Western society?

Please don't misunderstand me: there is an evolving and progressive literature base to support the use of probiotics when specifically considering gastrointestinal symptoms; it is just that they are not necessarily the ones currently being sold in our high street supermarkets.[7]

Coming back to testing for allergy, when I look at the available tests – whether York laboratories, Vega (electrodermal) testing, sputum tests for Candida, hair analysis and unknown serological testing – for which there is no conventionally reported validation, then there is a risk attached. The risk is this: you have got a medical problem or disease which has not been recognised or diagnosed yet and you may be embarking on a journey in the wrong direction. So please, please be careful about what you read and consider as valid. Of course many of my non-medical friends will say that is all very well but 'what if you go and see your doctor and he or she is not interested or dismissive or you have been through the conventional Western medical process and found it to be impersonal having come out the other end with no diagnosis'. 'What do you advise then?' they ask. That is the difficulty and I completely understand that. Every time I hear this question with that specific description of doctors, deep down I know there is truth to this description of some clinical consultations which may occur. Furthermore I then imagine someone somewhere saying exactly this about me. I am sure it will be true. So I don't have an easy answer for this and I have thought about it a lot because I see many patients who have come for a second and third opinion. My view is this. If you have gone through the conventional system and nothing has been found but you still have symptoms and are dissatisfied, seek a second conventional Western medicine opinion. If you have gone through the conventional medical system and nothing has been detected but you still have symptoms which concern you but are satisfied with the consultation and feel you have had the important diseases excluded, then make an appointment to discuss this with your doctor. Tell your doctor you are thinking about investigating complementary and alternative medicine: by doing this you are taking your physician with you. This is important as it is your passport back from 'No man's land'. Who knows, perhaps your physician may even come with you in this journey and learn about this practice of medicine for which we (people like me) have so little knowledge, but has been practised by alternative practitioners for thousands of years. I am not saying that every doctor will irreversibly shut their door to you if you seek an alternative or conventional medicine consultation, I am simply providing a framework to try and avoid this happening on those rare occasions.

Rule number 4 of Gluten Attack:

Primum non nocere, first do no harm to yourself and if you are unhappy with the medical advice you have been given seek a second opinion.

What is wheat allergy?

Given the definitions we have just discussed then I hope this is enlightening in terms of our understanding of wheat allergy. Wheat allergy is like the other IgE mediated food allergies. Yes, wheat is the culprit but that is where it stops in terms of bearing any resemblance to, for example, coeliac disease. Wheat allergy can be tested for using the conventional and validated methods I described earlier but once again with a supportive history. Both in the USA and UK it is in the top group of culpable antigens for IgE mediated allergy. Wheat allergy can present with food allergy, contact urticaria, atopy, eczema and respiratory allergy. Respiratory wheat allergy is due to inhalation of wheat flour and the proteins contained within; it is sometimes called baker's allergy for obvious reasons. Finally, wheat dependent exercise-induced anaphylaxis is rarely reported but does occur with the same features as I described for other food dependent exercise-induced anaphylaxis.

What is food intolerance?

We have now established our evidence base for food allergy. With these issues clarified let us discuss food intolerance. International population surveys have suggested up to 20–35% of society self-report symptoms when they eat specific foodstuffs which individuals have identified for themselves. This high prevalence has to be counter balanced against the 'gold standard test' of double blind placebo controlled food challenge. When this is applied then the prevalence of reactions related to food may fall to 2–4% – an almost ten-fold reduction! Top of the charts for self-reported symptoms are wheat based products, dairy products, caffeine and certain vegetables. The critical difference between food allergy and food intolerance is that food intolerance is not considered to have an immunological basis. This is the killer punch for medics, because there is no diagnostic test for food intolerance. This makes food intolerance very difficult to accept from the conventional Western medical perspective and thus falls into the realms of 'Bad Science'. How can we possibly make a diagnosis without a valid test? The only test which has been suggested previously are IgG antibodies. IgG antibodies have been reported to be implicated in food intolerance but are also present in the general population.

Symptoms for food intolerance overlap with food allergy. This includes gut symptoms, skin rashes, respiratory symptoms and then more non-specific symptoms like fatigue, headache, and musculoskeletal symptoms. Overlap with both Irritable Bowel Syndrome and fibromyalgia have also been reported. This association is something I would like to return to in Chapter 10. Doctors can discriminate between food allergy and food intolerance by assessing the history of the patient. Food intolerance is not considered to have the immediacy of food allergy with patients not reporting symptoms rapidly after exposure to the suspected food. There is said to be a prolonged symptomatic phase. Finally, and in my opinion crucially, the IgE serology test is negative in patients who are considered to have food intolerance. This currently makes food intolerance what I and others in the medical community would call a diagnosis of exclusion. The starting point is to exclude food allergy and then conclude that the patient has food intolerance with some supportive history.

So in the medical solar system of food allergy and food intolerance, two terms used interchangeably by society (like our New York waitress), doctors view them as entirely separate and different, with one being Neptune and the other being Mercury. No two planets could be further apart. One has a clear test, is recognised to be immunologically mediated and has an evidence base; the other does not.

There are a few anomalies to this, of which the first and most common is lactose intolerance. Dietary lactose is related to dairy products, in other words based on cow's milk. The enzyme lactase lives on the surface of the small bowel (which I described in detail on page 14). Lactose is a sugar and dietary lactose is broken down to smaller sugars, glucose and galactose, by the enzyme lactase operating from the small bowel surface. In essence when you drink milk it reaches the small bowel, our 'hot house' for absorption, and there it meets the lactase enzyme which allows it to be broken down to smaller sugars which can cross the small bowel barrier and be absorbed. Primary lactose intolerance is when you do not have enough lactase enzyme to process the milk you consume. The lactose does not get broken down and does not get absorbed. When the lactose reaches the colon (or large bowel) it gets broken down by bacteria that live in the colon (fermentation). Lactose also has an 'osmotic effect' – think of lactose being like a sponge absorbing water. The lactose draws water into the colon. This combination of fermentation and osmotic effect results in bloating, abdominal discomfort, increased wind and diarrhoea and once again can overlap with Irritable Bowel Syndrome type symptoms. Given this explanation I hope that it makes sense that if you have a shortage of this enzyme then the more milk you drink the more likely you are to get symptoms. What I have described earlier (page 26) as a dose-dependent response. Primary lactose intolerance is incredibly common and may be as high as 20% of the population. However, the development of symptoms is based on the interplay of how much enzyme you do or do not have and how much milk you consume.

Secondary lactose intolerance occurs in any condition which damages the small bowel surface. If you strip the lining of the small bowel then understandably as a consequence of this you do not have enough lactase enzyme. Thus any individual with a small bowel disease, for example undiagnosed coeliac disease, may have a secondary lactose intolerance.

Another anomalous example of food intolerance along very similar lines to lactose is fructose intolerance. Again fructose is a sugar absorbed in the small bowel. Unlike lactose it does not require an enzyme as it piggybacks a ride across the small bowel with glucose. Any unabsorbed fructose which reaches the colon plays out in exactly the same way as I have already described for lactose. Both lactose and fructose intolerance clearly differ from other food intolerances. They have a clear pathway for absorption and if you have a genetic predisposition or if this pathway is interfered with (like secondary lactose intolerance) this results in symptoms. Furthermore there are validated tests which can be used to diagnose these specific intolerances. Hydrogen breath tests can be used to diagnose these conditions. Breath tests are based on measuring the excessive hydrogen which we produce and exhale when our bacteria within the colon break down or ferment these sugars.

Bad Science, Bad Medicine or Bad Press

In the *British Medical Journal* article 'Bad Medicine: Food Intolerance', the author correctly asserts that there is an absence of evidence for food intolerance when assessed by contemporary Western medical standards. He also describes that a UK based charity, Allergy UK, receives funding from the food industry. He concludes 'Perhaps there is no harm in this food anxiety culture. But where will this dubious "free from" food fad lead? Food intolerance is being driven by profit and market forces, not medical forces, and this is always bad medicine.'[8] Personally I also think society has been voting with their feet and have embraced food intolerance but I appreciate that this may also be driven by market forces. I think it is really important for there to be medical debate about controversial issues where our medical practice is uncertain or there is an absence of evidence. Historically I would have been entirely in agreement with the final paragraph from 'Bad Medicine' which I have quoted. However, my own personal experience in recent years has been somewhat different and this has made my medical mind less polarised. **The question I keep asking is this: what if there is an association between food intolerances and symptoms but at present we just don't have the medical tool kit to recognise it?** I have had personal experience of this both with patients and the medical community when specifically considering the relationship between Irritable Bowel Syndrome type symptoms and coeliac disease. This is something which I will cover in detail in Chapter 5. For this reason I try to keep an open mind.

Rule number 5 of Gluten Attack:

The absence of evidence should not be used as proof of no effect.

So let's go all the way back to the 'Bad Press' and that New York waitress's 'is that health or lifestyle' question. I would like to try and answer that question. When I undertake the emergency work as a Consultant Gastroenterologist things are busy, emergency patients can be really sick and you may be up continuously through the night. Everyone doing emergency work or on-call is in the same boat. It is easy for tempers to get frayed. So I have a standard sentence I have trained myself to use when making referrals to other doctors on-call or asking for support from other medical colleagues (some of whom I don't always know). It goes like this: 'Hello, I am David Sanders, I am one of the gastroenterology consultants and I am on-call, can you help me?' I then go on to describe the patient, medical information and what my specific request is about. I find that sentence 'can you help me' is disarming and may defuse unnecessary exchange of unhelpful words which may occur in the heat of the moment. So what I would like to say in response to the waitress is this: 'Sorry can you help me? I am a person who suffers with coeliac disease, it is a disease process [emphasis gently on the word disease] which causes inflammation in my gut and makes me feel ill when I am inadvertently exposed to gluten. Please can you advise about what I am able to eat safely in your restaurant?' I hope that would alleviate the Bad Press and try and protect me from being 'glutened'; after all I know I have coeliac disease and I am at their mercy so to speak. I am really hoping this will get the best result.

I also hope that over the course of reading this book you may perceive that there is enough emerging evidence to have a similar view towards gluten sensitivity and if faced with this question you would be in a position to answer in a similar manner. I am hoping that if you have been diagnosed with gluten sensitivity, perhaps having a knowledge of the medical literature which I am describing within the course of these chapters may somehow empower you.

Finally an alternative! There is the devil in me that is incensed by this comment on the patient's behalf. In a parallel world I would like to say this: 'Thanks for asking me that question. Let me clarify this for you: coeliac disease is a disease that causes inflammation when I am inadvertently exposed to gluten. That is why it is called a disease. I may even develop symptoms while in your restaurant which would be unfortunate for you, me and all your other customers. So in answer to your question I think that is called health.' I know on my part that is neither Bad Press or bad medicine, just simply bad manners!

> **Rule number 6 of Gluten Attack:**
>
> Understanding the differences between wheat allergy, coeliac disease and food intolerance may help you manage your symptoms.

References

1. Karajeh MA, Hurlstone DP, Patel T, Sanders DS. Chefs' knowledge of coeliac disease (compared to the public): a questionnaire survey from the United Kingdom. *Clin Nutr* 2005;24:206-10.
2. Aziz I, Karajeh MA, Zilkha J, Tubman E, Fowles C, Sanders DS. Change in awareness of gluten related disorders amongst chefs and the general public in the United Kingdom: a 10 year follow-on study. *Eur J Gastroenterol Hepatol* 2014;26:1228-33.

3. Lis D, Stellingwerff T, Shing CM, Ahuja K DK, Fell J. Exploring the Popularity, Experiences and Beliefs Surrounding Gluten-free Diets in Non-Coeliac Athletes. *Int J Sport Nutr Exerc Metab* 2015;25(1):37-45.

4. Aziz I, Sanders DS. Patients who avoid wheat and gluten: is that health or lifestyle? *Dig Dis Sci* 2014;59(6):1080-2.

5. Turnbull JL, Adams HN, Gorard DA. *Aliment Pharmacol Ther* 2015; 41(1):3-25. doi: 10.1111/apt.12984. Review article: the diagnosis and management of food allergy and food intolerances.

6. Lomer MC. Review article: The aetiology, diagnosis, mechanisms and clinical evidence for food intolerance. *Aliment Pharmacol Ther* 2015; 41(3):262-75.

7. Gaisford S. Comparative survival of commercial probiotic formulations: tests in biorelevant gastric fluids and real-time measurements using microcalorimetry. *Benef Microbes* 2015;6(1):141-51.

8. Spence D. Bad Medicine: Food Intolerance. *BMJ* 2013;346:f529 doi: 10.1136/bmj.f529.

CHAPTER 5

Does Irritable Bowel Syndrome really exist and is there a link to gluten?

Heresy

Irritable Bowel Syndrome is very common; it is said to affect anywhere between 5–25% of the population depending on which criteria you use to define IBS. The origins of IBS date back as far as the 1940s in the medical literature and there have been more than 10,000 referenced medical publications on this subject. The first key issue surrounding IBS was how to make a diagnosis. Physicians back in the 1970s kept asking questions: how do we make a diagnosis of IBS? By doing this could we avoid putting patients with unexplained gastrointestinal symptoms through unnecessary investigations? A landmark study from the 1970s was by Adrian Manning who created criteria for making a positive diagnosis for IBS. This concept was something which was to be applied by gastroenterology doctors on patients who present to gastroenterology clinics with unexplained gastrointestinal symptoms. The importance of this study was the idea that by using fixed criteria two things could potentially be achieved. Firstly the patient was spared invasive endoscopic (camera) tests and a whole raft of other possible investigations. The second issue was that if you applied the criteria to your patients there should be no overlap with significant disease. For example, if you had undiagnosed Inflammatory Bowel Disease (IBD: a condition which causes inflammation in your bowel and can present with diarrhoea, blood in your stools and weight loss) and were presenting to a gastroenterology clinic with these symptoms and no diagnosis yet, then it was essential that the IBS criteria did not incorrectly identify and diagnose you as someone who had IBS when you should have been diagnosed with Inflammatory Bowel Disease. In time the criteria were refined many times over by experts in the field of IBS. We currently have the internationally accepted and established Rome III criteria for IBS:[1]

Irritable Bowel Syndrome

Diagnostic criterion*

Recurrent abdominal pain or discomfort** at least three days/month in the last three months associated with *two or more* of the following:

1. Improvement with defecation
2. Onset associated with a change in frequency of stool
3. Onset associated with a change in form (appearance) of stool

*Criterion fulfilled for the last three months with symptom onset at least six months prior to diagnosis.
**'Discomfort' means an uncomfortable sensation not described as pain.

In pathophysiology research and clinical trials, a pain/discomfort frequency of at least two days a week during screening evaluation is recommended for subject eligibility. www.romecriteria.org/criteria

Now you have had a chance to study the criteria I am sure that you will have noticed something very specific: there is no diagnostic test. No blood test, no biopsy to be looked at under the microscope to look for inflammation. IBS is a SYNDROME, a constellation of symptoms (as noted above) on which we base the diagnosis. This is amazing to me. The medical community have somewhere along the line accepted this as enshrined doctrine. Can you see a paradox here by comparison to the medical community's response to the more contemporary suggestion of gluten sensitivity? We have experts in IBS; extensive research in IBS; it is completely established within the medical community. In fact we specifically emphasise the importance of 'making a positive diagnosis for IBS'. We emphasise how important it is for IBS to not be a diagnosis of exclusion. This is to be discouraged and frowned upon as a clinical approach. 'Try to avoid unnecessary tests in these poor patients, let's not put them through all this indignity only to find nothing.' Of course there is extensive literature to support this approach but for me I have always been slightly troubled by this. IBS accounts for between 25% to 40% of a gastroenterology consultant's outpatient or office based physician's work load. It is a massive amount of our gastroenterology practice. The standard letter from primary care may say something like this: 'this lady has been coming to see us for some time with IBS but she is concerned that there may be something more, please can you see and advise her accordingly'.

Why would there be a difference in approach and acceptance between IBS and gluten sensitivity? Medicine, as I said in the Introduction, for me is neither a science nor an art: it is something in between. The medical wheels are slow to turn and more often than not this is in the interests of the patients and society as doctors are less likely to make mistakes by taking this cautious approach. The IBS model has stood the test of time. My only concern is that actually I could trace reports of gluten sensitivity dating back to the 1970s but, despite this, as yet it has never received the same medical recognition.

So let us come back to discuss the uncertainties which surround IBS. When it comes to therapeutic studies for IBS a variety of drugs have been trialled and there is a consistent pattern of a significant and large placebo effect. The placebo effect that I mentioned earlier is essentially an improvement in symptoms reported by the recipient of the drug even if it is an inert substance. Most clinicians would expect at least a 25% placebo effect for any drug study of IBS. Consistently there have been difficulties in providing significant symptomatic benefit for patients with IBS using conventional therapeutic drug models of treatment because the placebo effect is so large. Why is that? Perhaps it is because lots of the patients we see and diagnose or label with IBS don't actually have IBS? Maybe IBS is a diagnosis of exclusion and that there are a number of key conditions which we should exclude when patients present with IBS type symptoms? Perhaps I would dare to suggest that making a 'positive diagnosis' of IBS is exactly the wrong approach for the patients who we are seeing in our clinics? Please note that I am very specific in my terminology 'IBS type symptoms'. These patients may fulfil the Rome III criteria perfectly, they have IBS type symptoms but actually there is a diagnosis lurking within many of them waiting to be recognised. Imagine a circle with a 100 people with IBS type symptoms standing inside. Then imagine a battery of tests: with each set of tests we remove a group from the circle with a new diagnosis for their IBS type symptoms. The 100 within the circle get smaller and smaller. The circle is diminishing in size. Once these diagnoses have been excluded then we are left with a much smaller cohort of people within the circle that are negative for these tests. Now with this much reduced group size and having excluded a number of alternative diagnoses (for people who we said have IBS type symptoms) could I put forward my view that now we are left with true IBS? There is a subtle but important difference in terms of terminology between IBS type symptoms and IBS; this is because I would like to change the physician mind set. IBS type symptoms first presenting to a doctor do not need a positive diagnosis of IBS without investigation. They need their IBS type symptoms to be investigated thereafter; having done this, the physician can then conclude that they do indeed have IBS. Could I suggest that if we took this approach then the drugs that we consider so ineffective may be of great value as we would be treating the right patients? True IBS patients would get IBS treatments appropriately. Of course, as I said at the beginning, I am a medical heretic!

You and your microbiome – who is ruling who?

There is no doubt in my mind that there are certain IBS models that work very well. We know that we have microorganisms existing within our body as part of our natural state of health. The gut microbiome (sometimes called the gut flora) are residing primarily in the colon and have a role to play in terms of fermentation, gas production and therefore gastrointestinal symptoms. There has been much interest and research in the gut microbiome especially within the last 20 years. Currently it is considered that there are 100 trillion microorganisms in our intestine which is ten times greater than the total number of cells in our body (the mind boggles). The interesting theory which I have heard a number of lectures about is that perhaps the microbiome has an intimate relationship with its human host and that a change in the composition of our individual microbiome is the difference between the microbiome being a friendly part of our natural environment to becoming intimately involved in the development of a disease state. Such models with evidence of association have been demonstrated in Type 1 diabetes, multiple sclerosis, obesity, rheumatoid arthritis and even some models for cancer.[1] Some researchers have provocatively suggested that perhaps it is the microbiome that is in charge of us and not the other way around as we would like to believe! Let's jump to the outlandish parallel statement that Yuval Noah Harari (Professor of world history at the Hebrew University of Jerusalem) made, that wheat is running the show and mankind is a bit player who is present solely for the purpose of tending it (Professor Harari suggests this in his book *Sapiens: a brief history of humankind*, mentioned back in Chapter 1). Does that make you wonder?

The microbiome in patients with IBS has been shown to be different to that of healthy controls that do not have IBS. The models of post-infective IBS (developing IBS after a proven gastrointestinal infection) or IBS after a course of antibiotics (antibiotics given to a person for another reason) have been reported extensively and of course, in light of the information that we have discussed above, fits perfectly with the microbiome theory. Both gastrointestinal infection and systemic antibiotics alter our microbiome: some are killed and others proliferate in the absence of their fallen comrades. Thus IBS may follow. So please don't get me wrong. I am completely convinced by the data to support IBS as an entity to be diagnosed and treated appropriately and believe that there are proven scientific mechanisms for its development but I just want to remove the IBS type symptoms patients from this mixed bag of presenting symptoms before I treat those left with true IBS.

Her name was Betty

I worked for an inspirational boss without whom I would not have achieved anything. There are many of us who can say this in our professional careers. The difference for me was that Professor Bardhan was not just an intellectual inspiration but also a role model. He is a man of great modesty and humanity in what can be the very rough and tumble world of medicine. I imagine an investment banker reading this and laughing suggesting that there are far more terrifying professional worlds out there and I am merely ignorant and closeted. This may be true, nevertheless the traits I have described above are important when looking after people and can sometimes be forgotten or side-lined in my profession. Prof returned me to the values and principles which I had been taught by my parents but had perhaps forgotten along the way. Prof always said 'in every patient, if you listen there is a PhD'. In my case her name was Betty. It was 1998 and I was undertaking my clinic at the Royal Hallamshire Hospital (Sheffield, UK) just like any other working day. Betty had been referred to secondary care by her general practitioner for relatively longstanding gastrointestinal symptoms. These symptoms had come and gone over the years. Betty was in her mid-40s, she was a lady who worked as a full-time administrator and these symptoms were interfering with her professional life. She had light brown hair and had a slim build. At first meeting it was apparent to me that Betty was intelligent, articulate and polite. In the course of the consultation I documented that she fulfilled the Rome criteria for IBS. She told me that she wondered if she had coeliac disease. I sat back from my desk and pushed back a little in my chair. Betty explained her reasoning: she told me she had been doing some reading and investigation around these medical subjects. She told me that her family doctor had reassured her that she had IBS and that there was really no need for further investigations. To my shame I smiled. It is the kind of smile we have all seen on someone's face. I guess if I am honest it was a patronising smile; of course she had IBS, she fitted perfectly and by the way when did she get a medical degree and start making diagnoses? She could read all of this in my unspoken face. Betty gently said 'You are not going to test me for coeliac disease are you?' After some discussion I reluctantly agreed. Six weeks later Betty was sitting in front of me again. Her blood test done at that first meeting was positive. A positive endomysial antibody and her duodenal biopsy confirmed villous atrophy: she had a cast iron diagnosis of coeliac disease. When we next met she was far too gracious to gloat and I was too ashamed to have the courage to apologise. If you have ever watched the Jim Carrey movie *The Grinch* there is a scene in it where the Grinch is sitting in his cave contemplating and he shouts out loud in despair 'I am an idiot'. The echo he receives, which appears to come from the cave thinking for itself, is 'You're an idiot!' This was how I felt. We have met many times over the years, Betty and I, her symptoms resolved on a gluten-free diet. She and I both know the truth of our interesting journey together. In every patient there lies a PhD if you would just listen …

The first reported association between IBS type symptoms and coeliac disease

I took this single case experience to my colleagues and we discussed the whole sequence of events. The recurring question was 'could this be simply by chance alone?' Betty was a one off? After all we make a positive diagnosis of IBS based on fulfilling symptom based criteria. So I and my wonderful colleagues embarked on a journey. We prospectively undertook a study to see if there was an association between coeliac disease and IBS. Sequential unselected patients presenting to our secondary-care hospital were investigated for coeliac disease if they fulfilled the Rome II criteria for IBS (the Rome Criteria are periodically updated and at the time of our study it was the Rome Criteria II that were in use). We recruited 300 patients. Participants were initially investigated for coeliac disease with serum antigliadin antibodies and endomysial antibody. Any participant that had a positive antigliadin or endomysial antibody was offered a duodenal biopsy to confirm or exclude the diagnosis of coeliac disease. We demonstrated that coeliac disease was found to be present in 4.7% (14/300) of patients referred to secondary care fulfilling the Rome II criteria for IBS, a seven-fold increase compared to non-IBS matched controls (0.67%), (95% CI 1.6-28.0, p = 0.004). We were stunned, we knew it was previously unreported and that it would be ground breaking. The work was extensively presented in forums both nationally and internationally and finally in 2001 it was published in *The Lancet*.[2] I had a roller coaster ride with this novel observation many times. When I presented these data to the medical fraternity I would be extensively questioned. One particular incident I will recall to illustrate how hard it can be when your views are not within accepted medical doctrine of the time. This was a large audience by medical standards, more than 100 doctors in the room including some notable established and very well respected IBS researchers. After I finished presenting the data a senior academic gastroenterologist stood up in the audience and said two things: 'I have been undertaking research in IBS for years and I have never seen a case of coeliac disease, this is the first report and I am not sure I believe there is an association.' I wilted under scrutiny. The *Lancet* paper was accompanied by a similarly damning or indifferent editorial and so it continued in the international literature. Since that time there have been almost 20 studies which have broadly confirmed that preliminary observation. A recent systematic review and large meta-analysis (this is when we review all the published evidence and try to put the data into one mega dataset to see if we can see a clear relationship; it is viewed in scientific terms as very rigorous) found the prevalence of biopsy-proven coeliac disease in patients meeting the diagnostic criteria for IBS was more than four-fold that in control patients without IBS.[3] The recently published NICE guidelines stipulate that testing patients presenting with IBS type symptoms for coeliac disease is mandatory. The international gastroenterology medical community would now be shocked if you had not tested your IBS type symptoms patients for coeliac disease. In fact more often than not these days it is the family practitioner (general practitioner or office-based physician) that has done the serological test and is simply now referring for you to confirm the diagnosis by performing the gastroscopy and duodenal biopsy. The wheels of medicine have turned in one direction irreversibly all because of Betty. There was one sentence which I have heard many times over when listening to doctors: 'I don't believe in'. I have been given from a colleague an excellent response which I wished I had thought up for myself. Medicine is not theology: it is not for us to believe or not believe, we simply need to study the evidence and draw conclusions accordingly.

Since the coeliac disease–IBS association was published I and other colleagues have shown associations for patients presenting with IBS type symptoms and bile acid malabsorption, small bowel bacterial overgrowth and exocrine pancreatic insufficiency. Some of these associations are still viewed as controversial, there are still only a limited number of studies assessing the relationship, but the literature is evolving with time. More and more I hear clinicians suggesting that IBS should be a diagnosis of exclusion in order to not miss other associated diseases or conditions which may present with IBS type symptoms; perhaps I am not such a heretic after all!

It was a 10–15 year journey to change medical practice. I currently wonder if we are on the same journey for gluten sensitivity but perhaps an even longer timeline.

The Irritable Bowel Syndrome–gluten sensitive link

The provocative role of food in Irritable Bowel Syndrome

The public have for a very long time described that food can trigger gastrointestinal symptoms. Somewhere between 60–95% of patients with Irritable Bowel Syndrome have suggested that they either have specific foods which trigger symptoms or they report that their symptoms occur after eating a meal. Historically, this perception had initially some significant following in taking what is called an 'elimination diet' approach but was often termed the 'lamb, rice and pears diet'. This was highly restrictive but appeared to be very successful at improving symptoms when the researchers reported their findings. Why did this not become a mainstream intervention for patients reporting gastrointestinal symptoms related to food? There were two problems. Firstly, the degree of dietary restriction made adherence in the long term outside of a trial (or research) setting impractical and, secondly, the results were never particularly replicated by others in the field. However, this food–Irritable Bowel Syndrome link persists both in the general public's mind and some researchers'. A unique publication from 2013 further supports this view.[4] The investigators suggested that patients with Irritable Bowel Syndrome and food related symptoms had a higher burden of symptoms overall and worse quality of life than those Irritable Bowel Syndrome patients who did not report food related symptoms. So you can see that the hunt has always been on for a more specific food trigger. This of course leads us to the gluten story.

The first steps towards establishing gluten sensitive Irritable Bowel Syndrome

Sometimes when you publish research you emphasise a certain aspect to the research which seems novel but thereafter when you actually look back or look again at your data you may see another story hiding within all along. It may be something you missed at first sitting. It is a little like looking at some art where you are first drawn to looking at one aspect of beauty but then see something extraordinary which the artist has hidden within. A controversial example of this may be the suggestion that there is an image of a woman holding a child hidden within Da Vinci's *Last Supper*. Or if you look at Gustav Klimt's work of art *Judith* initially you see the amazing definition of the lady in question but if you look at the bottom right hand corner you realise that there is a man present in this picture, which in fact I believe is the clue to the real context and meaning of this painting.

At the same time that I published the controversial *Lancet* IBS study a group of German researchers published work looking at a coeliac-like appearance of patients who presented with IBS.

The German team investigated 102 patients presenting with diarrhoea and IBS type symptoms.[5] They described a sub-group of patients within the 102 who had features which made them resemble coeliac disease. The patients in this sub-group had the right HLA genetic association (DQ2 or DQ8). Some of them had an increased number of intraepithelial lymphocytes (the first attack cell of coeliac disease) on duodenal biopsy. They specifically did not have any evidence of villous atrophy. At the time of performing the gastroscopy (camera test) they sucked small bowel fluid through a channel in the gastroscope and when this was analysed in a laboratory, the fluid revealed coeliac antibodies in 30% of the cases they investigated. A similar finding was observed in the blood based antibodies. They suggested that a sub-set of patients presenting with IBS had a 'coeliac like' appearance. The investigators later published further work showing that if you had the HLADQ2 or DQ8 genetic association then this sub-group of IBS was more likely to respond to a gluten-free diet.[6] These were landmark studies. I read them and went back to my data set. I realised that 18% of my IBS study cohort had gliadin antibodies present although the duodenal biopsy was normal and thus excluded coeliac disease. Furthermore in my primary care study (which I discussed in Chapter 1) I had shown that although coeliac disease affected 1% of the 1,200 people I tested, a further 12% had a positive gliadin antibody but had normal duodenal biopsies. So to summarise, 12% of the general population have a gliadin antibody and 18% of patients with IBS have this gliadin antibody present in our reported data. What does this mean? It means that people are eating gluten; it is crossing their small bowel gut barrier and generating an immune response which results in the production of antibodies (which we can measure in our blood stream). It also suggests that if you have gastrointestinal symptoms you are more likely to have a positive antibody than if you are from the general population. When I went back to our data I realised that this perfectly complemented the German team's observations. Thus was born the first reports and suggestion of gluten sensitive Irritable Bowel Syndrome.

I tried in vain to get further funding to explore this; I cannot tell you how many charities and industrial companies I submitted my proposal or research grant to without having any success. Unfortunately that is the way research sometimes goes. The idea got placed in a drawer after I ran out of steam. One of the criticisms that may cause concern both to doctors and the general public about research is when there appears to be a link between the research findings and a funding party who may have a commercial interest in the results of the research. So you can see why the medical community will be concerned if Allergy UK is receiving funding from the food industry. Many would suggest that this is a conflict of interest. The problem is this: what do you do if you cannot get funding for your idea? Then you are very grateful if you find a commercial sponsor. This is always going to happen although the purist will say that is not acceptable. I would say the outcome of the 'black and white' approach to funding is this: put simply whole areas of medicine which are less emotive (in other words not children, cancer or the heart) from a societal perspective would not receive any funding. There would be no advancement of knowledge. Some data or information is better than no data as long as those involved conduct ethical studies and are transparent in showing their data and studies to others as well as declaring conflicts of interest, with for example commercial companies. Of course this is only my view and I am a pragmatist and not a purist, and maybe I am wrong.

Convincing the scientific community that gluten and IBS are linked?

The German study and our work are observational studies. In other words we undertook an intervention and then observed the effect. However, this type of study is not viewed as the 'gold standard' as I said earlier in Chapter 4. So what was really needed was a double blind placebo controlled food challenge; this was the level of evidence which I and others felt was required to convince the scientific community.

Little did I know that while I was working on this theory and trying to raise funding there were investigators on the other side of the world having exactly the same thoughts.

The FODMAP story

FODMAP stands for Fermentable Oligosaccharides, Disaccharides, Monosaccharides and Polyols, hence the acronym FODMAP. All saccharides are basically one form or another of sugar. So this is really a story all about sugar, how it is absorbed from the gut and whether sugars have the potential to cause gut symptoms. These FODMAP sugars have to be subdivided. Oligosaccharides comprise two groups, fructans and galacto-oligosaccharides. Disaccharides are typically lactose. Monosaccharides equate to fructose and then finally Polyols which are sorbitol, mannitol, maltitol, xylitol, poly-dextrose and isomalt. These sugars have two effects: first they may draw fluid into our bowel and secondly fermentation by gut bacteria (predominantly the bacteria in the colon) may lead to the production of gas (hence the F in FODMAP). These actions can be the route of gastrointestinal symptoms for some patients. It is important to clarify that these effects are not mediated through any immunological pathway. These sugars do not generate antibodies in people who have adverse reactions. So this is a non-immunological mechanism or you may want to consider this as food intolerance.[7]

The interest in FODMAPs is really a recognition that our westernised diet has changed over many years with an increased consumption of FODMAPs. FODMAPs are present in fruit (part of our five a day), concentrated fruit juices which exist in our fridge as a staple part of our diet and are consumed regularly at breakfast times with a view that this is one of our five per day. All positive messages of course and this may be the case for most of the general population but maybe not those who have gastrointestinal symptoms. Fructose (the monosaccharide) may be the biggest culprit because it is used extensively by the food industry. For example, high quantities of fructose are present in corn syrup which is a significant component in processed foods, ready to heat meals, soft drinks, yoghurts and bread.

The problem with FODMAPs is that they are poorly absorbed. Let me give you an example: glucose is not a FODMAP but it is the most basic sugar. Glucose is absorbed at the level of the small bowel in our bodies. After we consume any food or drink which contains glucose then our various enzymes try to break down what we have consumed to basic nutritional building blocks. Glucose is one of these building blocks and it is carried across the villi in our small bowel both by facilitated diffusion (a passive process) and by secondary active transport. I am labouring this point because for FODMAP sugars this does not apply. They are poorly absorbed and thus rattle through the small bowel, if you wish, and enter the colon where the majority of our gut bacteria live. Some FODMAPs such as fructose can hitch a ride and piggyback across our small bowel with glucose but this is not the case for the rest of the FODMAPs. Thus the more you consume the more present within your gut. The Australian group who have pioneered this work have sometimes called FODMAPs the 'fast food' for our gut bacteria. The colonic bacteria can rapidly break down FODMAP components to produce hydrogen, carbon dioxide and methane gas. This fermentation can then in turn lead to gastrointestinal symptoms and of course we must not forget the osmotic effect (drawing fluid into the bowel) which can lead to loose stool or diarrhoea. I like the idea of calling FODMAPs the 'fast food' for our gut bacteria because it also for me has a double meaning. I believe it is the processed foods which we eat that have a high FODMAP content and thus in some sense it is our own fast food habits which may have a role to play in our symptoms. Ready to heat versus cook it yourself, symptoms versus no symptoms? To complicate matters further some of the worst culprits may be things we do not think of as unhealthy, for example: mushrooms, garlic, onion and broccoli to name a few. Damned if you do, damned if you don't? Just being devil's advocate or provocative.

So where do you start when looking at what foodstuffs contain FODMAPs? There are a huge and diverse number of foodstuffs that do contain them, to varying degrees (see appendix). This is something

I will return to a little later. For now I would say that the Australian group provided a fascinating and progressive scientific story to support the role of FODMAPs in causing gastrointestinal symptoms in patients with Irritable Bowel Syndrome.

The first double blind randomised study of the effect of gluten in patients with IBS

The Australian group (led by Professor Peter Gibson from Monash University, Melbourne, an associate and international colleague) advertised in local newspapers and e-newsletters within metropolitan Melbourne that they were seeking to conduct a study looking at the effect of gluten on our gut and whether it could be the cause of gastrointestinal symptoms.[8] Participants who responded were eligible to take part if they were over the age of 16 years (i.e. an adult and not a child), fulfilled the Rome III criteria for Irritable Bowel Syndrome and had been investigated for coeliac disease but conclusively found not to have coeliac disease (in other words the wrong genetics, which virtually excludes coeliac disease or they will have had a gastroscopy with duodenal biopsy which was normal while on a normal gluten-containing diet). So in my opinion these were very rigorous inclusion and exclusion criteria. Finally the participants having fulfilled everything I have described above had to have self-reported that they noticed an improvement in their Irritable Bowel Syndrome symptoms when they placed themselves on a gluten-free diet. The participants were asked to collect information about symptoms and keep a food diary (again excellent dietary research study techniques) for two weeks prior to being given any intervention. This is what we call the run-in period where we look at baseline symptoms of participants before changing things for them. For example, during this time all participants continued on their self-imposed gluten-free diet (which they had described as working well for them in terms of improving their symptoms). The patients were then blindly randomised to either enter the placebo group or the gluten receiving group. The investigators had brilliantly created muffins which did or did not contain gluten. By the way these foodstuffs were also low in FODMAPs. The bread and muffins which participants were given either had no gluten in them (placebo group) or 16 grams of gluten in total. Remember earlier I mentioned that the average slice of bread is thought to have 2–3 grams of gluten. Following this intervention patients were followed up for six weeks during which time they continued on either the placebo or gluten arm. Both investigators and patients did not know which patients had been allocated to which arm of the study, placebo or gluten. So this was the double blind randomised gluten intervention study we had all been waiting for. So what did they find?

Thirty-four patients were recruited and completed the study protocol which I have described. In order to assess symptoms something called a visual analogue scale was used. Again this is a very well accepted and validated tool. You show patients a line with a score from 0 to 100 (or sometimes 0–10) and you ask them to put a cross at where they feel they score. So 0 may represent no symptoms and 100 may be the worst symptoms ever. Using this visual analogue scale the Australian team were able to demonstrate that after one week patients receiving gluten had far worse symptoms than those who were in the placebo group. If we step away from the whole concept of medical science and statistical significance what could we tell our patients based on this study? If you have Irritable Bowel Syndrome and have noticed that gluten may play a role in these symptoms then you are likely to be correct and using the gold standard of the double blind randomised controlled approach it appears that a gluten-free diet may indeed improve your symptoms. The size or magnitude of the difference for a patient who took part was that being on a gluten-free diet gave a 28% reduction in symptoms. In other words, of the patients who were given the placebo, 40% said they still had significant symptoms, compared to 68% in the group who received gluten.

Why is nothing ever straightforward in science!

The study I have described in detail was published with much fanfare; at last the scientific community had the evidence it required to recommend that a gluten-free diet was a good option with a firm evidence base in patients with Irritable Bowel Syndrome. Gastroenterologists like me across the world were delighted that the work had supported a view which we had suspected. Then things got a little more complicated …

Another wonderful friend, this time from Italy, published a very important study of more than 900 Irritable Bowel Syndrome patients.[9] Data had been collected over a ten-year experiment using the double blind placebo controlled approach but this time using not a gluten-free diet but instead a wheat-free diet. If you recall, gluten is within the endosperm of a wheat kernel but the other two components are the wheat husk and the embryo. So a gluten-free diet only excludes one aspect of wheat. The Italian group reported that 276 of the 920 patients were identified as being wheat sensitive (not far off a third) and those patients' symptoms deteriorated when given a wheat-containing diet. Once again the respected methodology of a visual analogue scale was employed. Interestingly the investigators categorised their wheat sensitive Irritable Bowel Syndrome patients into two sub-groups. One sub-group of the wheat sensitive IBS patients also reported multiple other food hypersensitivities (for example, cow's milk, eggs and tomatoes). Furthermore these patients were more likely to have a history of other atopic diseases, self-reporting symptoms related to wheat and a history of food allergy in infancy. So this sub-group you might say are more on the food allergy side of the IBS spectrum. For the second sub-group of the 276 patients who responded to a wheat-free diet there was a distinct 'coeliac-like' picture. These patients were more likely to have appearances suggestive of coeliac disease but not diagnostic. So they may have the right HLADQ2 or DQ8. They may have an increased number of intraepithelial lymphocytes on their duodenal biopsy or even a family history of coeliac disease.

So now gastroenterologists like me were in a quandary: was it the gluten or the wheat which was the culprit? What should we recommend to our patients, a gluten-free diet or a wheat-free diet? Should some patients be sub-grouped based on the Italian data into food hypersensitivity and others categorised as being coeliac like? I know how confusing this was for us at the time so I really hope I am not confusing you! It is really important for me to try and convey the fact that this is real science and real data. Sometimes when I look at reports about science the portrayal may be a rather unilateral headline grabbing statement. 'The cure to IBS is a gluten-free diet.' As you can see from reading these accounts and a description of the actual studies, a single magic bullet is never the case even if we would want it to be so. This is important because if you have symptoms like Irritable Bowel Syndrome it is essential that the perspective or medical counsel you are given is balanced and evidence based. It will allow you to have an understanding of the potential benefits you may derive if you were to go on a gluten-free diet, a perspective of the degree of benefit you may derive and finally an appreciation that there may be several ways to improve your symptoms and that if one fails then another may be worth trying. Managing expectation is a critical aspect of medical consultation and I believe the key to success and helping patients is to give them good evidence based counsel. They are then empowered both to understand what is being offered and also to make the decisions for themselves.

Wheat-free! Gluten-free! FODMAP-free! What's it to be?

So now I would like to introduce you to a third study! ☹ I hope you are hanging in there? The Melbourne group published a second data set.[10] They used the identical recruitment method (from their previous study) and again asked participants who had IBS type symptoms but with self-reported improvement on a gluten-free diet to take part. This time they used a much more specific dietary intervention. They did not just supplement the participants' diet with bread or muffins that were gluten containing or placebo, this time they provided all meals and thus completely controlled what patients were eating. This as you can imagine is considered to be even more scientifically rigorous. I could suggest to you that being absolutely sure if you are eating gluten or not is difficult at the best of times. You may buy something in good faith and it can contain gluten. So in the first Australian study I described then it would be possible for participants to inadvertently consume gluten while eating the food which they obtain for themselves unrelated to the bread and muffins supplements which they are given. In this second study by entirely supplying all food which participants eat you avoid this risk and of course the food supplied has the certainty of being gluten-free as dietitians are actively determining the food given to participants. This time there were three arms to the study, placebo, high gluten (16 grams per day) and low gluten (2 grams per day). The difference between their previous study and this current study which I am describing is that if you took part previously you were randomised to either getting gluten or not getting gluten (placebo). In this study all participants would go through each of the three arms of the study. So if you took part you would have one week on placebo, one week on 2 grams of gluten and one week on 16 grams of gluten. Of course you are randomised so you will not know in which order this is coming to you. Once again the participants had a two week run-in period at the start of the study during which time they were on a gluten-free and low FODMAP diet. What was observed in this study was that patients throughout the study irrespective of whether they got low gluten, high gluten or no gluten reported symptoms. The only time when patients were symptom free was in the two week run-in period at the start of the study when they were on a gluten-free and low FODMAP diet. So they concluded that their previous observation that gluten sensitive Irritable Bowel Syndrome exists was redundant and that their new results only showed benefit when patients were on a low FODMAP diet. How could the same investigators have two studies with such different findings and opposite conclusions? One reason may be what is called the nocebo effect. This is the opposite if you wish of the placebo effect. In the placebo effect you think an inert intervention is benefiting you. In the nocebo effect you think an intervention is causing you harm. Let us consider this from the perspective of people who took part in this study. In this study patients know for certain that when they take part they will be given gluten at some stage. In fact they will be given gluten for two out of the three arms that they will be put through (as they have to cycle through all three arms during the course of the study). In the previous study they knew that they had a 50% chance of avoiding gluten. However, in this study, patients who consider that they develop symptoms when they eat gluten report symptoms at a similar level whether or not they are having no gluten, some gluten or a lot of gluten. Why? They are anticipating harm as a result of the study design. This is the nocebo effect.

So suddenly what we had hoped was clear water has become very muddy again with conflicting studies. What I have done is to summarise the published FODMAP literature in Tables 1 and 2, below. This will give you I believe a picture of the uncertainty within the field. I would then like to try and make sense of the data from taking an overall approach.

Table 1. Summary of FODMAP studies

Country	Year	Patients (N = number of patients)	Outcome
Australia	2006	N = 62 Uncontrolled	74% Response Rate to FODMAP diet
Australia	2008	N = 25	The reintroduction of fructans to the patients caused symptoms in >70%
Australia	2010	N = 30	The reintroduction of fructans to the patients caused significant symptoms
Australia	2010	N = 34 self reported gluten sensitive IBS	Significant reduction in overall symptoms in GFD group
UK	2011	N = 82 IBS randomised	76% response on a FODMAP diet but for those who received standard dietary advice rather than specifically a FODMAP diet – there was still a 54% response!
UK	2012	N = 41 IBS randomised	68% response versus a 23% response for standard dietary advice
Norway	2012	N = 79 & N = 35 Healthy Subjects (Retrospective)	Significant Improvement in Pain
Australia	2013	N = 37 with IBS on GFD and/or FODMAP	Throughout the study patients had symptoms except at the beginning when the patients were only exclusively on a FODMAP diet. This period before a study starts is sometimes called the 'run in period'.

Country	Year	Patients (N = number of patients)	Outcome
New Zealand	2013	N = 90 Prospective Uncontrolled	72% satisfied with symptom improvement
Norway	2013	N = 46 Prospective Uncontrolled	Improvement in total symptoms
Switzerland	2013	N = 312 patients with a functional GI disorder	Of the 76% who completed the study there was adequate relief in 93%
Denmark	2014	N = 19 IBS patients	Patients documented a benefit (using a scoring system) on being on a FODMAP diet
Australia	2014	N = 30 IBS	~ 50% reduction in symptoms
Sweden	2014	N = 82 IBS	Equal response to FODMAP diet (56%) versus Traditional Dietary Advice (52%)

Table 2. Summary of Irritable Bowel Syndrome, gluten effect (and on one occasion wheat) and non-coeliac gluten sensitivity intervention studies

Country	Year	Patients (N = number of patients)	Outcome
Germany	2001	N = 102 IBS-D without CD	Stool frequency significantly improved in patients with HLA DQ2/DQ8
Germany	2007	N = 145 IBS-D without CD	HLA-DQ2 predicted response to GFD
Australia	2010	N = 34 self reported gluten sensitive IBS	Significant reduction in overall symptoms in GFD group (same study as described in the FODMAP Table 1)
Italy	2011	N = 920 patients with IBS	More than a third of the patients were responded to a wheat free diet
USA	2012	N = 45 IBS-D	Increased gut permeability in patients receiving gluten
USA	2013	N = 45 IBS-D	Reduction in stool frequency in patients on GFD
Australia	2013	N = 37 self reported gluten sensitive patients with IBS on GFD and/or FODMAP	All patients responded to reduction in FODMAPs during run-in period but no difference between GFD and gluten containing arms (same study as described in the FODMAP Table 1)

Country	Year	Patients (N = number of patients)	Outcome
Iran	2015	N = 72 patients	Significant improvement in symptoms for 84% of patients receiving the gluten-free sachets versus 26% for those patients being given gluten containing sachets
Italy	2015	N = 59 patients with self-reported Non-Coeliac Gluten Sensitivity	Double Blind Placebo Controlled challenge using gluten. Patients receiving gluten reported significant increase in symptoms
Italy	2015	N = 35 patients with Non-Coeliac Gluten Sensitivity	Double blind challenge inducing symptoms in only 1/3rd of the patients who thought they had symptoms related to gluten
UK	2016	N = 40 IBS-D	Significant improvement in symptoms with 72% of patients continuing gluten-free diet even at 18 months after the study finished

Confused and making sense of what doctors tell us?

I think what the two tables tell us is that there is active interest in this field with many of the studies being very recent. More importantly I might assert that there is much to be said on both sides of the debate. Whether you think it is gluten or FODMAPs and let's not forget wheat! So if the doctors are confused what can the poor patient do! There are a few points that I would like to make which may help our clinical approach. As you can see in the appendix, foods which contain FODMAPs are diverse and capture a large number of food groups. The initial recommendation is that you follow a strict low FODMAP diet for two months. Thereafter you need to go through a reintroduction period. The reintroduction should be done with one FODMAP at a time. Each reintroduction or challenge should be for one week. All of this should be done with careful dietetic supervision (the same applies in my opinion to a gluten-free diet or a wheat-free diet). So the FODMAP diet is both very restrictive and complicated. However, if you can identify which FODMAP group is causing symptoms you may subsequently find things far less restrictive. A gluten-free diet is not as restrictive, furthermore the food industry has clear markings for what is and what is not gluten-free. Finally in our own Sheffield, UK study (Table 2) we have shown that patients benefit even in the long term and at 18 months more than 70% are still committed to the gluten-free diet out of their own choice. Although I recommend dietetic support (and firmly believe this is the optimal medical care) some patients may want to get on and try and help themselves and a gluten-free diet in those circumstances may be an easier place to start. When I reviewed the Melbourne, Australia literature, on careful reading and scrutiny I discovered that most of the patients in the FODMAP versus gluten-free studies ultimately opted for a gluten-free diet at the end of the study period and of their own free volition. The patients said that they 'felt better' on a gluten-free diet.

Fructans are the oligosaccharides which I mentioned earlier and are considered part of the FODMAP family. Fructans are present in wheat; they are part of the wheat which is not linked to gluten. So in actual fact the whole medical debate may be somewhat semantic as FODMAP, gluten and wheat may all have some commonality. They are all dietary cousins! So what is a patient or clinician to do? I think the clinical approach is based on each individual patient. If a patient comes presenting with symptoms related to the consumption of gluten – they may be correct! The doctor needs to exclude coeliac disease and if there are any features that are like coeliac disease (coeliac lite I like to call it and you will see why in a moment!), then they may benefit from a gluten-free diet. The patient may be classified as having non-coeliac gluten sensitivity, or wheat sensitivity or be called patients who avoid wheat and gluten depending on whichever term is currently in fashion. If a patient presents with Irritable Bowel Syndrome and has not complained of symptoms related to eating gluten then they may still benefit from a dietary intervention. The selection of gluten-free, wheat-free (in effect a more stringent gluten-free as you are avoiding not just gluten but the other forms of wheat) or FODMAP can be based on careful history taking, investigation (for coeliac lite features) and discussion with the patient regarding which dietetic option they want to try first. If there are no coeliac lite features they may want to hit things hard and go down the FODMAP route. Alternatively they may think that they would rather start with the more straightforward (and well delineated in shops) gluten-free diet and if it does not work then ramp up to the FODMAP. After all, hopefully I have provided the evidence such that you can see the level of effect is not dissimilar, they are all dietary cousins and this then brings things down to personal choice. I told you I like my cola cans and I have tried to illustrate this in the figure below. It took me hours to draw so I hope you like it! Figure 1.

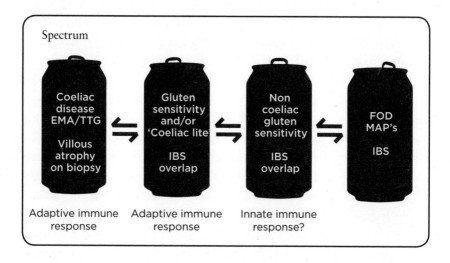

I really feel that this field of the Irritable Bowel Syndrome gluten sensitive link has moved forward significantly and to the benefit of patients. I hope I have convinced you of this and a belief that there are many approaches to the dietary management of IBS. This for me gives great hope to patients with IBS. We have come a long way from lamb, rice and pears. When I give this talk I always conclude by saying 'ladies and gentlemen, nutritional therapies for irritable bowel syndrome are at last back on the menu!' Having read this chapter I hope you feel the same way too?

References

1. Simrén M, Barbara G, Flint HJ, Spiegel BM, Spiller RC, Vanner S, Verdu EF, Whorwell PJ, Zoetendal EG; Rome Foundation Committee. Intestinal microbiota in functional bowel disorders: a Rome foundation report. *Gut* 2013;62(1):159-76.

2. Sanders DS, Carter MJ, Hurlstone DP, et al. Association of adult coeliac disease with irritable bowel syndrome: a case-control study in patients fulfilling ROME II criteria referred to secondary care. *Lancet* 2001;358(9292):1504-8.

3. Ford AC, Chey WD, Talley NJ, Malhotra A, Spiegel BM, Moayyedi P. Yield of diagnostic tests for celiac disease in individuals with symptoms suggestive of irritable bowel syndrome: systematic review and meta-analysis. *Arch Intern Med* 2009;169(7):651-8.

4. Böhn L, Störsrud S, Törnblom H, Bengtsson U, Simrén M. Self-reported food-related gastrointestinal symptoms in IBS are common and associated with more severe symptoms and reduced quality of life. *Am J Gastroenterol* 2013;108(5):634-41.

5. Wahnschaffe U, Ullrich R, Riecken EO, Schulzke JD. Celiac disease-like abnormalities in a subgroup of patients with irritable bowel syndrome. *Gastroenterology* 2001;121(6):1329-38.

6. Wahnschaffe U, Schulzke JD, Zeitz M, Ullrich R. Predictors of clinical response to gluten-free diet in patients diagnosed with diarrhea-predominant irritable bowel syndrome. *Clin Gastroenterol Hepatol* 2007;5(7):844-50.

7. Rajilić-Stojanović M, Jonkers DM, Salonen A, Hanevik K, Raes J, Jalanka J, de Vos WM, Manichanh C, Golic N, Enck P, Philippou E, Iraqi FA, Clarke G, Spiller RC, Penders J. Intestinal microbiota and diet in IBS: causes, consequences, or epiphenomena? *Am J Gastroenterol* 2015;110(2):278-87.

8. Biesiekierski JR, Newnham ED, Irving PM, et al. Gluten causes gastrointestinal symptoms in subjects without celiac disease: a double-blind randomized placebo-controlled trial. *Am J Gastroenterol* 2011;106(3):508-14.

9. Carroccio A, Mansueto P, Iacono G, et al. Non-celiac wheat sensitivity diagnosed by double-blind placebo-controlled challenge: exploring a new clinical entity. *Am J Gastroenterol* 2012;107(12):1898-906.

10. Biesiekierski JR, Peters SL, Newnham ED, Rosella O, Muir JG, Gibson PR. No effects of gluten in patients with self-reported non-celiac gluten sensitivity after dietary reduction of fermentable, poorly absorbed, short-chain carbohydrates. *Gastroenterology* 2013;145(2):320-8.

CHAPTER 6

How does gluten attack?

Is there any evidence that gluten can attack people who do not have coeliac disease?

I f you recall in Chapter 1 I described the immunological pathway of attack for gluten in patients that have coeliac disease when they are exposed to gluten. This was a specific immune mediated response. I also suggested in Chapter 3 that our own published work corresponded with other international investigators; we were all reporting a high prevalence for the genetic HLA association of DQ2 or DQ8 when we were seeing patients who presented by self-reporting symptoms related to eating gluten. Table 2 in Chapter 5 gives you a plausible explanation for this appearance which suggests similarities to coeliac disease, the 'coeliac lite' picture which we are collectively recognising in our patients. So is non-coeliac gluten sensitivity just a lesser form of coeliac disease? Or given the absence of a clearly defined blood test or disease marker, is non-coeliac gluten sensitivity actually a form of food intolerance? Could it be unrelated to gluten but instead it is actually another component of wheat or even FODMAPs that is the culprit? These questions led to a group of international investigators meeting in 2010 to discuss our views and try and reach a consensus.[1] First we reviewed two small studies trying to look at how gluten attacks in patients who do not have coeliac disease but do have symptoms reported when they consume gluten. What was observed was that an inflammatory response occurred but that this was as a result of an alternative immune system to the one described in coeliac disease.

In patients with coeliac disease it is our adaptive immune system which creates a response to gluten. The adaptive immune system is all about recognition of a new 'pathogen', for example gluten, and then evolving immunological memory of this event so that if re-exposed you have a defence system primed and in place. The studies showed that conversely patients with non-coeliac gluten sensitivity did not have this adaptive immune response in the same manner as coeliac patients but instead their reaction was via a different part of our natural immune system also called the innate immune system. The innate immune system is again involved in defence from any pathogens (a typical example would be against bacteria) but there is no stored memory after the event. Perhaps we could consider that the innate immune system is a more generic or non-specific defence. Nevertheless the emerging work from these small studies suggested that the innate immunity could be the culprit in non-coeliac gluten sensitivity patients. Thereafter two further novel observations have been made. Firstly, there was a suggestion that a particular component of wheat may be implicated, the amylase trypsin inhibitors (ATIs). Amylase trypsin inhibitors are plant derived proteins. Their biological role is to stop the effect of attack enzymes from common plant parasites, for example mealworms which have an appetite for wheat. ATIs are present within the endosperm and are also potent stimulators of the innate immune system. The ATIs can drive production of the immune soup which then causes inflammation. This theory and the emerging evidence would fit perfectly with the non-coeliac gluten sensitive patients. It also provides an immune pathway which is unique and distinct from coeliac disease.

More recently an international collaboration of investigators has attempted to directly visualise changes in the small bowel in real time.[2] The team used a technique called confocal endoscopy. I have previously described conventional endoscopy in Chapter 3. The only difference with confocal endoscopy is what is at the tip of the scope. A conventional endoscope magnifies what we look at by approximately x 50 while confocal magnification is at the level of more than x 1,000. The views are so amazing when looking at the surface of the bowel that the term has been coined real time histology. In other words in real time you can directly see what is happening on the surface of the bowel as if you had taken a sample and sent it off to a pathologist for microscopic dissection and analysis. The technique is currently a research tool. The investigators recruited 36 patients with Irritable Bowel Syndrome and suspected food intolerances that were willing to participate. They placed the confocal endoscope into the small bowel looking directly at the villi. They then directly administered diluted food antigens through another portal within the endoscope. This meant that the injection of diluted food antigen landed straight onto the surface of the small bowel. This bypasses the need for the patients to eat the food and partially digest it. Within five minutes of exposure to the diluted food antigens the small bowel in real time showed a significant increase in the number of one of its favourite attack cells, the intraepithelial lymphocytes. Also as the inflammation occurred the surface of the small bowel started to open up, develop leaks and create pathological spaces between the villi. This happened in 61% (22/36) of the cases they tested and the commonest food antigen to give this response was? You guessed it: wheat, the three others being cow's milk, yeast and soya.

So for me there is emerging evidence that gluten has a direct role in attacking the small bowel. The means of attack is the subject of on-going research but we are seeing some kind of signal from independent research groups. The Gluten Attack appears to be unrelated to the path that we recognise in patients with coeliac disease. Of course further work is required but this is exciting! Do you remember the question I posed about food intolerance in Chapter 4?

'The question I keep asking is this: what if there is an association between food intolerances and symptoms but at present we just don't have the medical tool kit to recognise it?'

Makes you think?

How do I know if gluten is attacking me?

This is a simple question really; the vast majority of patients I have seen have identified gluten for themselves. The international consensus group (of which I am part) have worked on creating a hit list of

Table 1. Characteristic appearance (phenotypes) of self-reported NCGS in adults[3]

Female prevalence: 72–84%
Mean age: 30–40 years old
Lower gastrointestinal symptoms
Diarrhoea: 16–54%
Constipation: 18–24%
Altered bowel habit: 27%
Abdominal pain/discomfort: 67–83%
Bloating: 72–87%
Weight loss: 25%
Upper gastrointestinal symptoms
Upper abdominal pain: 52%
Nausea: 9–44%
Inadvertent swallowing of air (Aerophagia): 36%
Gastro-oesophageal reflux: 32%
Mouth ulcers (Aphthous stomatitis): 31%
Extraintestinal symptoms
Skin rash (eczema or dermatitis): 6–40%
Brain: depression 15–22%; foggy mind 34–42%; anxiety 39%; confusion 5%; headaches 22–54%
Limb numbness: 6–32%
Joint or muscle pains (fibromyalgia-like symptoms): 8–31%
Fatigue: 23–64%
Lack of well-being: 68%
Data taken from several reports. Abbreviation: NCGS, non-coeliac gluten sensitivity.

symptoms and I have added some further aspects based on our experience of an extensive group of patients with non-coeliac gluten sensitivity. To tell you the truth the patients know this better than we do and were able to advise and guide accordingly.

How do we diagnose non-coeliac gluten sensitivity?

I think the first issue is to see if your symptoms fit? If they do then the second and really important question is whether you have been tested for coeliac disease. Critically if you have been tested then ask yourself, when you had the blood test or the camera test were you on a self-imposed gluten-free diet. If you were the test is null and void. Now I have already discussed the importance of the HLADQ2 and HLADQ8 genetic association in patients with coeliac disease in Chapter 1. Suffice to say if you are on a gluten-free diet and you have not had tests for coeliac disease then one option is having your HLA gene status checked. HLADQ2 or DQ8 genes account for virtually all cases of coeliac disease. However, this genetic pattern is present in 25–40% of the general population. This means the test can only be used to exclude coeliac disease. If you are negative for HLADQ2 or DQ8 genes it is very unlikely that you will have coeliac disease. If you have the HLADQ2 or DQ8 association then you fit within 25–40% of the population. You may have coeliac disease but remember only 1% of the population have coeliac disease although the presence of the right HLA is much higher. This of course brings us to the dreaded gluten challenge! This is something I discuss with patients regularly. Understandably if you have identified that gluten makes you ill and are on a gluten-free diet then it is very hard to go back in time to clarify the diagnosis. I have discussed this extensively in Chapter 1. Put simply, best to clarify the diagnosis at the outset. However, the real world is not like this and we are human. So what does a gluten challenge involve? Conventionally it requires more than 10 grams of gluten (four slices of bread) per day for 6–8 weeks. This is very poorly tolerated. After that period you have your gastroscopy with biopsies looking for villous atrophy (evidence of coeliac disease). You also have your antibodies checked looking for the positive blood tests I mentioned earlier in this book: endomysial antibody or tissue transglutaminase antibody. Recent work may improve our ability to perform this test in clinical practice. A landmark American study revealed that over 75% of patients with coeliac disease will demonstrate changes on the duodenal biopsy after 3 grams of gluten for only two weeks. This is so much more tolerable for patients. My own clinical experience is what I call the rule of thirds. One-third say 'never ever am I undergoing a gluten challenge', one-third try the gluten challenge and develop awful symptoms rapidly (we have to stop the challenge early and perform their gastroscopy and biopsy) and the final third manage to get through the whole challenge. This involves careful counselling, timing for the patient (to fit with their professional and life commitments) but ultimately the patients I have seen are glad for the clarification of which group they fit into: coeliac or non-coeliac gluten sensitivity.

So this is the journey that faces anyone who is reading this book and wonders if they may have symptoms related to gluten or if gluten is attacking them. There may be other indicators for individuals at the time of diagnosis (if they have not placed themselves on a gluten-free diet). We and others have reported a high prevalence of the gliadin antibodies. These gliadin antibodies are, however, non-specific and cannot be used as the deal clincher to make the diagnosis of non-coeliac gluten sensitivity. The presence of gliadin antibodies may just point us in the right direction. Symptom response is also a very useful clinical indicator (as long as coeliac disease is excluded at the outset).

A single patient's personal journey

Let us look at the case of Andrea. Andrea is 54 years old and runs her own business. In her shop there are critical peak spells of high customer footfall, generally lunchtime and the end of the day, but she also has steady customer business throughout the day. Andrea advises people about which glasses they should wear or buy. There are some aspects of measurements and technical detail which can be challenging. Over the last six months she had noticed progressive difficulty in concentrating or what she described as having a 'foggy mind'. She had been to see her family doctor who checked for all the important and common conditions such as anaemia or an under-active or over-active thyroid. She was coincidentally noted to have an increased frequency in her bowel habit. She was given a probable diagnosis of Irritable Bowel Syndrome, reassured and things were left open for further review if necessary. Andrea became convinced that food was playing a role in her symptoms. She read extensively and tried to cut out lactose initially without benefit. She then read about a gluten-free diet and experimentally tried this for a few weeks. She felt there was an improvement and went back to see her family doctor. Andrea was advised that she could have coeliac disease and referred. When I first met Andrea after discussing her history which I have already described with gentle questioning she told me that she had carefully picked her appointment time because her symptoms are worst in the morning and after eating. She had also never mentioned that on a few occasions 'she had been caught out in the shop'; she became tearful at the embarrassment and shame which she felt on recounting this. She confided that she had worn a continence pad to attend the appointment today. She had in recent times been avoiding social events because of feeling 'not in control'. During the day she found giving advice about specifications of the glasses she was selling were sometimes 'hazy' and she 'looked like an idiot', she said. She felt this was impairing her ability to advise her customers in a professional manner.

We went through the gene tests, gluten challenge and also a colonoscopy. These tests were all normal. Andrea saw our expert dietitian and was given advice about a gluten-free diet based on the history, exclusion of coeliac disease and clinical diagnosis of non-coeliac gluten sensitivity. When Andrea saw me four months after this her symptoms had resolved. She felt like a 'new person'. Her stool was formed and she had control. She had not had any episodes of incontinence, urgency or soiling for more than two months. Her mind no longer felt 'clouded'. She had previously not mentioned joint pain in predominantly her hands but this had also improved. Of her own volition she continues on a gluten-free diet. I know this is only one case history but I can say that I have now seen more than 200 such cases with different and very personal stories. The international research community within my field is also reporting a similar experience.

References

1. Fritscher-Ravens A, Schuppan D, Ellrichmann M, et al. Confocal endomicroscopy shows food-associated changes in the intestinal mucosa of patients with irritable bowel syndrome. Gastroenterology 2014;147(5):1012-20.e4.
2. Sapone A, Bai JC, Ciacci C, Green PHR, Hadjivassiliou M, Kaukinen K, Rostami K, Sanders DS, Schumann M, Ullrich R, Villalta D, Volta U, Catassi C, Fasano A. Spectrum of Gluten-Related Disorders: Consensus on New Nomenclature and Classification. *BMC Med* 2012;10(1):13.
3. Catassi C, Elli L, Bonaz B, Bouma G, Carroccio A, Castillejo G, Ciacci C, Cristofori F, de Magistris L, Dolinsek J, Dieterich W, Francavilla R, Hadjivassiliou M, Holtmeier W, Korner U, Leffler D, Lundin K, Mazzarella G, Mulder C, Pellegrini N, Rostami K, Sanders DS, Skodje I, Schuppan D, Ullrich R, Volta U, Williams M, Zevallos V, Zopf Y, Fasano A. How the Diagnosis of Non-Celiac Gluten Sensitivity (NCGS) Should Be Confirmed: The Salerno Experts' Criteria. *Nutrients (in-press June 2015)*.

CHAPTER 7

Sheffield, centre of the gluten universe!

There, I have said it in the title of this chapter. It's embarrassing I know to make such an arrogant proclamation. So what is this arrogant man talking about?

In Chapter 8 you will hear all about my wonderful friend and beloved colleague Professor Marios Hadjivassiliou. He is a Professor of Neurology and THE world expert on neurological aspects of gluten related disorders. Now this is no idle claim. He has had an extraordinary research journey spanning 20 years during which time he trail-blazed the path which so many have followed since. It can only be described as a struggle which truly demonstrated the difficulties faced by any researcher and medical scientist who makes a unique observation. When you stand alone the noise of a crowd can drown you out, even if you are right. I will tell you more of his story later. So how can I substantiate my claim? Over the 20 years we have published more than 150 publications on gluten related disorders which I suspect is more than any other international unit. Marios brought a group of like-minded researchers together and launched the Sheffield Institute of Gluten Related Disorders (SIGReD).

I told you that I liked history and the surprises it throws up. After years of doing gluten related research I discovered an important paper. History taught me a lesson. Here we were, working as an internationally recognised group of researchers who we believed had raised the flag for gluten related problems and many would say put Sheffield on the world map for this medical problem, but there was someone before. In 1986 the first gluten-free versus gluten-containing study for schizophrenia was undertaken – where? You guessed it: the University of Sheffield, long before Marios or I had even turned up and started banging the drum![1] So even more evidence to support my claim for Sheffield!

Sheffield is the fifth largest city in the United Kingdom with a population of 500,000–600,000. Its deep industrial roots and labour traditions underpin the unique people of Sheffield. Following the end of the industrial revolution Sheffield blossomed into one of the greenest cities in the world. There are said to be more trees in Sheffield than any other city in Europe. The city is infiltrated everywhere with beautiful green tracts of land, parks or woods. The good people of Sheffield have made their city a city of sport, outdoor pursuits and students. I am lucky to call it home.

My father-in-law was an inspirational and internationally recognised paediatric urologist and he used to love to gently tease me. He lived in north-west London and he would say 'No one in the world knows Sheffield! So when you are going all over the world giving your talks don't say you are from Sheffield, say you are David Sanders from Sheffield London, then the whole world will know your name!' I would like to think he inspired me to try and advertise the beauty of Sheffield. I regularly feature aspects of the history of Sheffield whenever I am asked to speak about our medical research whether in the UK or internationally. I hope when you have read this section you will place Sheffield on your list of things to do or places to visit: if you do I promise you will not regret it.

Reference:

1. Vlissides DN, Venulet A, Jenner FA. A double-blind gluten-free/gluten-load controlled trial in a secure ward population. *Br J Psychiatry* 1986;148:447-52.

CHAPTER 8

The neurological effects of gluten; does gluten affect our behaviour and mood?

Establishing the link between coeliac disease and neurological disease

This chapter as much as anything charts the clinical career and research journey of my colleague Professor Marios Hadjivassiliou (Professor of Neurology at the Royal Hallamshire Hospital and University of Sheffield). It has been a fascinating journey to watch as a bystander and I learnt about two things beyond the science. The first was about my friend's tenacity and the second was about what I will term 'medical ideology'. The second issue I will come back to a little later. So let's talk about Marios. Like many talented people you meet I find recurrently if they excel in one domain then it is possible to do the same in another. Here is an example. As I said earlier in Chapter 7 Marios is THE expert in neurological manifestations of gluten sensitivity but he is also an excellent cook. There is no need when staying in Sheffield to eat at any of our fine local and ethnic restaurants: just ask the taxi driver to take you to the Hadjivassiliou household for a Michelin star culinary experience! Perhaps Marios' love of cooking also travelled into his profession given the work he has done in the field of gluten and neurology.

The first case reports of a relationship between neurological symptoms and features of malabsorption were described in the medical literature in 1966. The patients described were known to have coeliac disease. These patients were malnourished, had significant weight loss, low albumin (an important protein in our body which falls during starvation or malabsorption) and multiple vitamin deficiencies. The general consensus at that time was that the malabsorption led to the vitamin deficiencies that in turn led to neurological problems. The link between vitamin deficiencies and nerve damage is very well established. For example a low vitamin B12 level has been reported as a cause of nerve damage in our limbs (a condition described as peripheral neuropathy).

In 1996 Professor Hadjivassiliou produced a seminal paper entitled 'Does cryptic gluten sensitivity play a part in neurological illness?' Looking at gluten sensitivity from a neurological perspective Marios and his colleagues investigated patients with neurological disorders of unknown cause for evidence of sensitivity to gluten (using the then available blood test looking for the presence of gluten antibodies). They were able to show that up to 54% of neurology patients had such antibodies when compared to only 12% of the local healthy blood donor population. After doing the small bowel biopsies on all their neurology patients with positive antibodies they found evidence of coeliac disease in 16% (compared to 1% of the healthy local population). It was clear from this study that the commonest neurological problems linked to coeliac disease were ataxia and peripheral neuropathy. A second paper followed on defining and naming the condition when manifesting with ataxia as 'gluten ataxia'.[1] Marios had gathered the largest number of patients with unexplained ataxia ever reported with this problem. Ataxia is a neurological term which reflects problems with walking and co-ordination of movement in arms and legs. Your balance is affected and because people feel unsteady they walk with their legs apart (you may or may not have heard of the term broad based gait); this spreads their body mass over a wider area and makes it less likely that they will fall. Patients with ataxia may also experience problems with clumsy arm movements and slurring of speech. You will know this because you can become ataxic (transiently) or unsteady with alcohol and historically if you are asked to walk a straight line 'heel to toe' by UK or USA police you know you are in trouble!

Ataxia can occur if the part of your brain called the cerebellum is damaged. The cerebellum is at the back of your brain and deals with balance. Further signs of cerebellar damage include your eyes moving in an uncontrolled fashion from side to side (nystagmus), a tremor of your hands, particularly when you are trying to pick up something, and slurred speech.

Over the course of his epidemiological studies Marios saw hundreds of patients (more than 1,300 when I last looked) in his specialist ataxia clinic. He showed that the presence of gliadin antibodies was high in these patients and that many of them (70%) also had the right HLADQ2 or DQ8 which is consistent with individuals who have coeliac disease. Now Marios confirmed the historical reports that some of the patients he was seeing had coeliac disease. He performed duodenal (small bowel) biopsies and demonstrated a flat bowel. He also showed that 60% of the patients with gluten ataxia had evidence of cerebellar atrophy (a loss of cerebellar tissue) on their Magnetic Resonance Imaging (MRI) brain scans.

Making the link to gluten sensitivity

The next step he took for me was crucial, completely novel and I think has helped many patients as well as changing our clinical practice internationally. Marios hypothesised that patients who did not have evidence of flat bowel but did have the positive blood test were still gluten sensitive and he offered them a gluten-free diet. When following up these patients he used the validated International Co-operative Ataxia Rating Scale to demonstrate that for those patients who adhered to the gluten-free diet there was significant improvement by comparison to the patients who chose not to try the diet. One of the other observations was that a gluten-free diet was more successful early in the disease than if you have had neurological symptoms for more than 12 months. This may be due to irreversible neural (nerve) cell damage which unfortunately can be the nature of progressive neurological diseases if untreated.[2]

Now this is not a randomised study I hear you say and I accept that but it is difficult to go back in time and undertake such a study. The observations were made over 20 years of follow-up and careful study. It is difficult, when faced with a patient who is getting worse with neurological symptoms that may be irreversible, to consider randomising patients to receive or not receive a gluten-free diet. There are significant ethical considerations. Think how you would feel if you were in the no gluten-free diet arm of the study and I had told you what I knew so far based on the published literature. Would you take part? This is not like Irritable Bowel Syndrome where the symptoms will persist or not depending on your intervention. With neurological symptoms there is progression and worsening which may be irreversible if there is a delay in treatment. We should perhaps not forget that the original observations by Dicke on the 'deleterious effect of gluten on children with coeliac disease' was indeed a published observation and not a result of randomised, controlled, double blind diet. Yet this is the historical evidence which resulted in us treating patients with coeliac disease with a gluten-free diet and is undisputed by the medical profession to this day.

Gluten related neurological disease and autoimmune process?

Marios has gone on to try and reveal the mechanisms behind the damage caused by gluten in these patients. He has shown loss of cerebellar tissue with lymphocyte infiltration (invasion of the tissue by white cells) of the brain in post-mortem studies of patients with gluten ataxia. He has described a specific tissue transglutaminase TTG 6 which appears to be present in patients with neurological gluten sensitivity by comparison to the TTG 2 which is typical in coeliac disease and the TTG 3 which is seen and considered specific for dermatitis herpetiformis.

One of the interesting features of coeliac disease is that deposits of anti-TTG antibody can be shown on small bowel biopsy. This has also been shown in other organs or tissues outside of the small bowel such as within the liver or muscle. Marios showed these deposits in the blood vessels present within the brains of neurological gluten sensitive patients. So these observations fly in the face of what was historically thought to be the cause of neurological damage in these patients. The theory of vitamin deficiencies as the primary cause of nerve damage looks less likely and the evidence for an autoimmune process is more convincing. Once again it appears that the gut is the entry point and then the autoimmune process determines which organ is affected.

Professor Hadjivassiliou has shown that gluten may also play a role in other neurological diseases and not just ataxia. His work in gluten neuropathy is equally convincing. There have also been reports for myopathy (muscle damage), encephalopathy and a rare condition called stiff man syndrome. Other investigators have reported a specific link between a form of epilepsy and coeliac disease. This type of epilepsy typically reveals calcified areas in the brain on imaging and is seen in younger patients.

The white matter (encephalopathy) story

We are all familiar with the term 'use your grey matter' which is equivalent to 'use your brain'. The brain is comprised of both grey matter and white matter. It is described in this way because of its naked eye appearance. Now the grey matter is thought to deal with brain function but white matter is much more about communication between different parts of the brain. White matter has never really been given the same status of importance as grey matter. However in 1988 the term of white matter dementia was first described. This was the idea that damage or loss of white matter could have a significant effect on our cognitive ability.

Marios and his colleagues had already anecdotally thought that patients with coeliac disease had far more neurological symptoms (including headaches) than were historically reported but they went on to show that MRI brain imaging revealed damage of white matter tissue in patients with coeliac disease.[3] Other investigators have validated these observations and even suggested that specifically in patients with coeliac disease there is an association with mild impairment of cognition. Patients may term this 'brain fog'. An Australian research group has shown in a small pilot study of 11 coeliac patients that their cognitive performance improved considerably after 12 months on a gluten-free diet by comparison to their baseline state at the time of diagnosis (when they were cognitively assessed but had not commenced a gluten-free diet).[4] So these are the first tentative steps towards a relationship between our mental function and gluten. This I think is the next challenge for researchers in the field of neurological gluten related diseases.

Here is a conversation I have had with many gastroenterologists which reflects 'medical ideology'.

Comment: 'I don't believe in neurological manifestations of coeliac disease.'

I ask: 'Why not? Have you read the published literature?'

Response: 'No, it's just that I have seen lots of cases of coeliac disease but very few with neurological symptoms or signs.'

I ask: 'Have you actually asked patients with coeliac disease about neurological symptoms or examined them?' Silence.

Comment: 'No, but I still don't believe in it.'

(Now imagine me inwardly screaming in despair.)

The problem is that we are all like this. I am like this! I wish I was not but I also behave like this in some aspects of my life. In fact I think we all do. We have beliefs which we hold dear and they are not always substantiated. So that is human nature but when it comes to medicine and looking after patients that can be a problem.

> **Rule number 7 of Gluten Attack:**
>
> If you have unexplained neurological symptoms then knowing whether you have positive gluten related antibodies or coeliac disease is important.

The brain–gut axis

This is an area of great controversy, uncertainty and interest. I would like to tread with great care. To be honest I think that the brain is the least understood organ in our body. Comparatively something like the heart or gut is so much better understood. Why is brain medical science not as advanced? One thing for sure, it is not for want of trying! There have been and are many amazing neurological, psychological and psychiatric investigators and scientists giving their professional lives to this field. The problem (and this is really a personal opinion) is that the brain is more complex than the other organs. At the end of the day I could suggest that the heart is nothing more than a pump and the gut is a tube which absorbs things along the way. What is the brain? Is the brain our very own and personal consciousness and the keeper of our own existence?

For some time investigators have put forward the theory of the brain–gut axis. The leaky gut allows some proteins to cross which would normally not be given a visa into our bodies! The proteins make it across our gut barrier and then into our blood stream; when they reach the brain they meet an important control mechanism called the 'blood–brain barrier'. Having made it across the gut barrier these proteins do the same in the brain. This then results in our immune response being activated within the brain which may be pathological and thus cause us abnormal symptoms, mood or behaviour. What proof can I give you of this? Intestinal permeability studies are a means of demonstrating holes within our gut (leaky gut). In order to do this we use sugars that we give the patient to drink (lactulose mannitol test). Lactulose is a large sugar and would not normally make it across the gut barrier but if there are a large number of holes then they can cross far more readily. These sugars are then absorbed by our bodies into our blood stream and then what happens to these specific sugars is that some are excreted. We get rid of some of them once they have been absorbed by us. We excrete them through our urine. So if we have a leaky gut then we will see an increased urinary excretion of these specific sugars when we take part in this test. Investigators have reported that more than 40% of children with autism spectrum disorders (ASD) and more than 35% of patients with schizophrenia have an increased urinary sugar excretion when using the intestinal permeability test.[5]

The gluten–brain effect?

When specifically considering the gluten effect, animal model studies have made some intriguing observations. Serotonin is a monoamine neurotransmitter and you may be familiar with the antidepressant class called SSRIs or selective serotonin resorption inhibitors (fluoxetine, paroxetine and such drugs from the same family). So serotonin in our brains is very important in terms of behaviour and cognition. Laboratory based investigators have demonstrated that giving rats gluten to eat may lower brain concentrations of something called tryptophan. Tryptophan is a precursor of serotonin and is necessary to produce serotonin. Thus the absence or reduction of tryptophan may ultimately lead to lower brain serotonin levels. We can then speculate that if the same thing occurs in humans when they eat gluten this may be the cause of the impaired cognitive function which has been reported.

There are other mechanisms which have been suggested. Gluten when partially digested is said to break down to an 'opiate- or opioid-like protein'. The term for this gluten opioid is called a gluten derived 'exorphin' and again in rodent models this has been shown to have a cerebral effect. The term opioid- or opiate-like will clearly indicate to you what sort of effect it may have on us.

Finally, do not underestimate the evolving belief that the brain–gut axis is a two way street. The brain may influence the gut and vice versa. The consumption of gluten will result in a certain gut microbiota pattern, or another way to look at this is that introducing gluten into the diet of humans who have not eaten gluten before will alter their gut microbiota. Very recent brain imaging studies have assessed the effect in humans over four weeks who have been given probiotics. The investigators showed that after four weeks of probiotics key areas of the brain involved in the processing of emotion or sensation looked differently on brain imaging compared to at the start of their study.[6] This technique of functional brain imaging was initially used to map which areas of the brain have control over which functions of our body but this radiological science has progressed. In this study the investigators are trying to demonstrate whether certain stimuli (for example, a probiotic) can have a particular effect on the brain. So the suggestion I am making is that if probiotics can have such an effect on the brain (working through the alteration of the gut microbiota) then it would not be a huge leap to imagine gluten having the same effect, although this work has never been done.

What evidence is there for mood and behavioural changes in non-coeliac gluten sensitivity?

Thirty-one patients with non-coeliac gluten sensitivity (in whom coeliac disease had already been excluded) were asked to eat four slices of white bread for three days. These patients were compared to healthy volunteers in terms of their responses to the ingestion of gluten. At the beginning of the study patients with non-coeliac gluten sensitivity had a higher baseline level of both anxiety and depression than controls. The consumption of gluten did not appear to make this situation better or worse.[7]

However, more recently the same Australian group who undertook the FODMAP research also reported a randomised placebo controlled double blind crossover study to look at this very issue.

I know you are thinking 'what type of study!?' Please refer to Chapter 1 for a detailed breakdown of the components of a study. The only additional thing here that I have not mentioned is the crossover component and this is exactly what it says: crossover means that patients take part in both limbs of the study and are crossed over during the study to make sure this occurs. Twenty-two patients known to have IBS but in whom coeliac disease had been excluded volunteered to take part. These were patients who had reported that even if they did not have coeliac disease they still noted an increase in gastrointestinal symptoms related to eating gluten. The patients were given three days of either 16 grams of gluten or 16 grams of whey protein, or not given any supplement at all. All patients crossed over to each of the three limbs of the study. The key finding was that when these individuals were given gluten they scored highly for depression which was not the case when they were given whey. The investigators concluded that this was the first study to demonstrate that short-term exposure to gluten induced feelings of depression.[8] Clearly there is more work to be done in this area but this study and the animal model work I described earlier may be used in tandem as the beginning of the body of evidence to support the negative effects of gluten on mood.

The controversy surrounding autism spectrum disorders, schizophrenia and the gut

I mentioned earlier that intestinal permeability studies have demonstrated increased permeability in specific conditions such as autism spectrum disorders and schizophrenia. The enteric nervous system or gut autonomic nervous system housekeeps for our gut and is involved in both movement (peristalsis) of the gut and gut permeability. Our gut has many nerve endings within it involved in control and these comprise the enteric nervous system. This system leads out to the vagus nerve. The vagus nerve has a direct communication with the brain. Thus the gut and brain are able to directly communicate. When mice are fed a particular lactobacillus (or good bacteria) they display reduced anxiety and depression behaviour. Fascinatingly if the vagus nerve is cut in these mice then even when the mice are fed the good bacteria it has no effect. It has no effect because there is no communication to the brain. The communication highway no longer exists. Furthermore germ-free mice (that have not been exposed to the normal germs and are reared in a sterile environment) also show abnormalities of the enteric nervous system. So this could be used to suggest that if a similar sequence of events occurred in humans this could result in a central nervous system disease process. The hypothesis works along these lines: in early life abnormal exposure to bacteria within the gut can result in increased intestinal permeability which then results in abnormal communication to the brain. This communication may cause cerebral inflammation and may be the basis for such conditions as autism or schizophrenia.

In autism spectrum disorders, opioid proteins have been implicated in causing abnormal central nervous activity. The two key opioid peptides are gliadomorphin and casomorphin which can be derived from eating wheat or milk respectively. A healthy gut which does not leak or have holes will not allow these peptides to pass, therefore it follows that a leaky gut allows absorption. This is described as the opioid theory for ASD. A gluten-free and casein-free diet (GFCF) has been shown to reduce intestinal permeability in children with ASD. This clearly supports the theory but the data showing the benefit of this dietary approach on behaviour is less clear. A randomised double blind crossover study of 13 children with ASD who were given either GFCF or placebo (six weeks for each) was unable to show any significant difference in behaviour whether these children were receiving GFCF or placebo.[9] This study also reported that parents could not determine whether the children were on placebo or GFCF. A second important study looked at 72 ASD children with 38 on a GFCF diet and 34 on a normal diet.[10] After 12 months there were highly significant differences in terms of improved social interaction, reduced degree of inattention and reduced hyperactivity in ASD children who were on the GFCF diet. The criticism of this positive study was that although there were 38 ASD children at the beginning of the study on a GFCF diet and 34 on a normal diet, by the end of the study the numbers were 29 and 26 respectively. This 'drop out' may affect the results. The study was also criticised for not using a placebo diet. The suggestion is that if parents know whether their child is receiving a normal diet or a GFCF diet then this may affect their responses about how their child is responding. For example, if you believe that a GFCF diet works perhaps you are more likely to see signs of it working or report that it works during the study. A systematic review of the studies published in this area has concluded that there is as yet insufficient evidence to advocate this dietary approach to children with ASD. This is an area where parents and families of children with ASD have a difference of opinion to the currently held medical perspective. Let me say again, this is an area of great controversy, uncertainty and interest. I would like to tread with great care.

Historical case reports or series have suggested that schizophrenia has an association with undetected coeliac disease and increased intestinal permeability. Recent American data has suggested a gluten sensitive link. In a study of 1,401 patients with schizophrenia the investigators showed a higher presence of gliadin antibodies (23%) by comparison to 900 controls (3%).[11] The team also showed that 5.6% of their schizophrenic patients had a raised TTG level by comparison to 0.8% in their control population. The investigators went on to report some symptomatic benefit to patients who were given a gluten-free diet.[12]

Other investigators have shown that Anti-*Saccharomyces cerevisiae* antibodies (ASCA) are raised in both patients with established schizophrenia and those who have recently developed schizophrenia.[13] ASCA may be viewed as a marker of gastrointestinal inflammation. The same team analysed their data further and were able to show that patients who had received anti-psychotic treatment had reduced ASCA levels by comparison to those schizophrenic patients that had not yet received treatment. This could indicate that the gut barrier or leaky gut integrity is improved when schizophrenic patients are treated with antipsy-chotic medication (which has a central and cerebral effect). So we could perhaps agree that this provides support to what I asserted at the beginning of this chapter, that the brain–gut axis is a two way street. Here is evidence of a treatment of the brain closing down holes in a leaky gut.

I would conclude by suggesting that these two novel data sets provide some evidence of a gut–brain barrier relationship and warrant further study.

References

1. Hadjivassiliou M, Gibson A, Davies-Jones GA, Lobo AJ, Stephenson TJ, Milford-Ward A. Does cryptic gluten sensitivity play a part in neurological illness? *Lancet* 1996;347(8998):369-71.

2. Hadjivassiliou M, Sanders DS, Grunewald RA, Woodroofe N, Boscolo S, Aeschlimann D. The neurology of gluten sensitivity. *Lancet Neurol* 2010;9(3):318-30.

3. Currie S, Hadjivassiliou M, Clark MJ, Sanders DS, Wilkinson ID, Griffiths PD, Hoggard N. Should we be 'nervous' about coeliac disease? Brain abnormalities in patients with coeliac disease referred for neurological opinion. *J Neurol Neurosurg Psychiatry* 2012; 83(12):1216-21.

4. Lichtwark IT, Newnham ED, Robinson SR, Shepherd SJ, Hosking P, Gibson PR, Yelland GW. Cognitive impairment in coeliac disease improves on a gluten-free diet and correlates with histological and serological indices of disease severity. *Aliment Pharmacol Ther* 2014; 40(2):160-70.

5. Julio-Pieper M, Bravo JA, Aliaga E, Gotteland M. Review article: intestinal barrier dysfunction and central nervous system disorders – a controversial association. *Aliment Pharmacol Ther* 2014;40(10): 1187-201.

6. Larsson MB, Tillisch K, Craig AD, Engström M, Labus J, Naliboff B, Lundberg P, Ström M, Mayer EA, Walter SA. Brain responses to visceral stimuli reflect visceral sensitivity thresholds in patients with irritable bowel syndrome. *Gastroenterology* 2012;142(3): 463-72.

7. Brottveit M, Vandvik PO, Wojniusz S, Løvik A, Lundin KE, Boye B. Absence of somatization in non-coeliac gluten sensitivity. *Scand J Gastroenterol* 2012;47(7):770-7.

8. Peters SL, Biesiekierski JR, Yelland GW, Muir JG, Gibson PR. Randomised clinical trial: gluten may cause depression in subjects with non-coeliac gluten sensitivity – an exploratory randomised clinical study. *Aliment Pharmacol Ther* 2014.

9. Elder JH, Shankar M, Shuster J, Theriaque D, Burns S, Sherrill L. The gluten-free, casein-free diet in autism: results of a preliminary double blind clinical trial. *J Autism Dev Disord* 2006;36(3):413-20.

10. Whiteley P, Haracopos D, Knivsberg AM, Reichelt KL, Parlar S, Jacobsen J, Seim A, Pedersen L, Schondel M, Shattock P. The ScanBrit randomised, controlled, single-blind study of a gluten- and casein-free dietary intervention for children with autism spectrum disorders. *Nutr Neurosci* 2010;13(2):87-100.

11. Cascella NG, Kryszak D, Bhatti B, Gregory P, Kelly DL, Mc Evoy JP, Fasano A, Eaton WW. Prevalence of celiac disease and gluten sensitivity in the United States clinical antipsychotic trials of intervention effectiveness study population. *Schizophr Bull* 2011;37(1): 94-100.

12. Jackson J, Eaton W, Cascella N, Fasano A, Warfel D, Feldman S, Richardson C, Vyas G, Linthicum J, Santora D, Warren KR, Carpenter WT Jr, Kelly DL. A gluten-free diet in people with schizophrenia and anti-tissue transglutaminase or anti-gliadin antibodies. *Schizophr Res* 2012;140(1-3):262-3.

13. Severance EG, Alaedini A, Yang S, Halling M, Gressitt KL, Stallings CR, Origoni AE, Vaughan C, Khushalani S, Leweke FM, Dickerson FB, Yolken RH. Gastrointestinal inflammation and associated immune activation in schizophrenia. *Schizophr Res* 2012;138(1): 48-53.

CHAPTER 9

The skin effects of gluten

The skin–gut connection runs along very similar lines to the brain–gut axis which I have discussed earlier. Some clinicians suggest that there are certain dermatological diseases where in order to heal the skin you need to heal the gut. Again we come to the concept of a 'leaky gut' which allows antigens that we eat to get across the small bowel. The concept here would be that this is not normally possible to the same extent in a healthy individual. Once across our small bowel the food antigen may stimulate an inappropriate immune response which can manifest itself through the skin.

A recent example of a skin–gut connection is a study which reported a connection between small bowel bacterial overgrowth and acne rosacea. The investigators studied 113 rosacea patients and 60 control patients without acne. They used the glucose hydrogen breath test to look for small bowel bacterial overgrowth and demonstrated that this was present in 46% (52/113) of the patients. Small bowel bacterial overgrowth only occurred in 5% of controls (3/60). Some researchers suggest that the breath test is not the most accurate test to reveal bacterial overgrowth of the small bowel but I would describe it as the best of a poor selection of tests that we currently have available. Nevertheless the researchers in this study I am describing went one step further to demonstrate the connection by actually treating these rosacea patients with rifaximin. This is an antibiotic which works specifically in the gut (it is not absorbed). The investigators asked all 52 patients with acne who were positive for small bowel bacterial overgrowth to take part in a randomised controlled study. They randomised 48 of the 52 patients who were willing to take part to either rifaximin for 10 days or placebo. The investigators then showed that after 10 days of antibiotic therapy with rifaximin the skin lesions cleared in 20 of 28 patients and greatly improved in 6 of 28 patients, whereas patients treated with placebo remained unchanged (18/20) or worsened (2/20). This was a highly statistically significant result. Placebo patients were subsequently switched to rifaximin therapy, and bacterial overgrowth was eradicated in 17 of 20 cases. Thereafter 15 of these 20 patients also had improvement or resolution of their skin symptoms. So the message is clear: there is a relationship between the gut and the skin when considering acne rosacea and this is revealed by a high presence of small bowel bacterial overgrowth in these patients. Treatment with appropriate antibiotics greatly improves skin symptoms in the majority of acne rosacea patients who have coexisting small bowel bacterial overgrowth.[1]

Are there any specific links between gluten and the skin? The best model for this theory is coeliac disease and a rare skin condition called dermatitis herpetiformis (DH) which I mentioned earlier in Chapter 1. Patients with coeliac disease are more likely to have skin related problems such as mouth ulcers, alopecia or vitiligo. Some of these features are a manifestation of being an autoimmune disease and thus have a higher risk of developing other autoimmune diseases. The autoimmune link may account for vitiligo and alopecia but for the mouth ulcers this may be driven by vitamin deficiencies that are common in patients with coeliac disease at the time of diagnosis.

DH is an uncommon itchy rash presenting with blisters typically on the buttocks, elbows, knees and sometimes your head. It was discovered that this skin condition had a unique relationship with coeliac disease.[2] If you take a small bowel (or duodenal) biopsy from patients with DH then >70% will have the flat bowel of coeliac disease but the other 30% will have the right genetics for coeliac disease and perhaps the presence of the initial attack cells, the intraepithelial lymphocytes (IELs), I mentioned earlier, in the absence of villous atrophy. Thus it could be argued that all DH patients have coeliac disease or early coeliac disease. If you biopsy the skin of patients with DH you can actually demonstrate the presence of tissue transglutaminase 3. This is so specific that it is used as a diagnostic test for DH. Furthermore this skin condition is treated by a combination of drugs and a gluten-free diet. So I consider the gut to be the point through which gluten 'breaks and enters', thereafter in patients with DH, for whatever reason, they then trigger a different immune response which then results in such patients presenting with this problematic skin rash rather than coeliac disease per se.

There have been claims (particularly on the internet) that other forms of dermatitis and eczema are affected or frequently reported after gluten exposure. However, the only disease which has been clearly studied is psoriasis. A Swedish dermatology research group suggested that for patients with psoriasis who have coexisting antigliadin antibodies (IgG or IgA) there may be a dermatological benefit to trying a gluten-free diet.[3] The investigators performed a case–control study involving 33 patients with psoriasis who were gliadin antibody positive and the controls were six gliadin negative psoriasis patients. The investigators tried to exclude coeliac disease in 31 of the gliadin antibody positive psoriasis patients by demonstrating a negative endomysial antibody (in all but two cases). Bear in mind that a positive endomysial antibody is the most predictive antibody of coeliac disease with a likelihood of having subsequent villous atrophy on duodenal biopsy which is greater than 90%. Interestingly although these psoriasis patients did not have villous atrophy some individuals did have increased duodenal IELs (15/31). After a three-month period on a gluten-free diet the gliadin antibody positive cohort showed a notable improvement in the psoriasis affected areas and this was also demonstrated using a validated severity index score for psoriasis. Of course there was also a reduction in these patients' gliadin antibody levels. This improvement was not seen in the gliadin negative cohort. When a gluten-containing diet was recommenced there was a deterioration of psoriasis in just over one-half of the gliadin positive patients. So this could suggest that in carefully selected psoriasis patients who have a positive gliadin antibody, their skin disease may benefit from a gluten-free diet. I have enthusiastically presented this Swedish study to UK dermatologists and understandably was told that this was a standalone study which requires further studies and validation. What I wonder about is why no one has ever tried to replicate this work or advance this area of research although this study was published in 2000!

So I think I would conclude by saying there is firm and accepted evidence of a relationship between DH and the value of a gluten-free diet but beyond this there remains uncertainty in the dermatological medical community. The internet tells me that the public are far more convinced than perhaps doctors are. I would love for there to be a new medical champion who tries to take the psoriasis–gluten link further, either to prove or disprove this claim once and for all, for the benefit of the psoriatic patient community. Of course I am of no consequence in this debate and am not even a dermatologist!

References

1. Parodi A, Paolino S, Greco A, Drago F, Mansi C, Rebora A, Parodi A, Savarino V. Small intestinal bacterial overgrowth in rosacea: clinical effectiveness of its eradication. *Clin Gastroenterol Hepatol* 2008;6(7):759-64.
2. Fry L, Keir P, McMinn RM, Cowan JD, Hoffbrand AV. Small-intestinal structure and function and haematological changes in dermatitis herpetiformis. *Lancet* 1967;2(7519):729-33.
3. Michaëlsson G, Gerdén B, Hagforsen E, et al. Psoriasis patients with antibodies to gliadin can be improved by a gluten-free diet. *Br J Dermatol* 2000;142(1):44-51.

CHAPTER 10

Are there links between gluten and fibromyalgia, myalgic encephalomyelitis or postural orthostatic tachycardia syndrome?

M yalgic encephalomyelitis or Chronic Fatigue has long been considered to have an association with coeliac disease. Like IBS type symptoms there has been a suspicion that patients with Chronic Fatigue type symptoms may have underlying undiagnosed coeliac disease. For this reason most guidelines for Chronic Fatigue recommend testing new patients with coeliac serology. Furthermore when Chronic Fatigue patients are questioned for coeliac associated symptoms there appears to be substantial overlap of the two conditions' symptoms. Recent work has even suggested that, in patients who try an exclusion diet as a means of improving their symptoms, a gluten-free diet is a popular choice. There remains to be any randomised studies as yet but clearly the door is open for such an approach.

The work done in fibromyalgia is both limited (with really only two studies) and intriguing. Very recently a series of 20 fibromyalgia patients were placed on a gluten-free diet. This particular group of patients had longstanding and quite disabling fibromyalgia symptoms. An important aspect of the study was that the investigators only suggested or instigated a trial of a gluten-free diet after conventional therapies failed. Coeliac disease was excluded by negative tissue transglutaminase antibodies or the absence of villous atrophy on a duodenal biopsy. Once again an increased presence of lymphocytes in the small bowel biopsy was reported in this carefully selected group of patients. After commencing the gluten-free diet the clinical responses of these patients were documented. All patients reported remission of fibromyalgia based on pain criteria. Some patients said they were now able to return to work. In some cases patients described themselves as returning to normal life or being able to stop opiate drugs which they had been medically prescribed for pain. The reintroduction of gluten was followed by a recurrence of their fibromyalgia symptoms.[1]

Another study builds on the first report I have described. This type of study is called a case–control study. You study the effect of an intervention between two groups, the case group and the control group. The investigators evaluated the effects of a gluten-free diet in 97 patients with fibromyalgia and coexisting IBS. Building on the previous mention of increased intraepithelial lymphocytes on the small bowel biopsy, in this case there were 58 fibromyalgia patients who had raised duodenal IEL and 39 had normal duodenal biopsies. So in this study the cases were patients with fibromyalgia (coexisting IBS) and raised IEL count on a duodenal biopsy while the controls were patients with fibromyalgia (coexisting IBS) and a normal IEL count on duodenal biopsy. The coeliac blood tests were all negative. At the beginning of the study all the patients were asked about symptoms. The patients with a high IEL count on biopsy (case group) recorded similar poor quality of life and high fibromyalgia and IBS related symptom scores compared to those fibromyalgia patients who did not have any increase in IELs on their duodenal biopsy (control group). After one year on a GFD, all outcome measures markedly improved by 26–30% in the increased duodenal IEL case group compared with 3–4% in the control group (who had a normal duodenal IEL count). These results stress the potential role of gluten as a trigger for the clinical manifestations of IBS and fibromyalgia. The study also suggests that increased duodenal IELs might be a useful clue to identify those patients who potentially benefit from gluten withdrawal.[2] The raised IEL count in fibromyalgia patients who appear to respond is intriguing and worthy of further comment. It is possible that these carefully selected patients may have had the early stages of coeliac disease or 'coeliac lite' given that a substantial proportion were HLADQ2 and/or HLADQ8 positive and showed increased duodenal IEL on their biopsy. Certainly to me it suggests that gluten exclusion may be worth trying in fibromyalgia patients who have failed conventional therapies and have any features to suggest they fall into the 'coeliac lite' group.

Postural tachycardia syndrome

Postural tachycardia syndrome (PoTS) is a group of disorders related to autonomic dysfunction.[3] The autonomic nervous system is involved in the housekeeping of our body. It helps maintain our blood pressure when we stand up so we don't feel dizzy. You may have heard of the term postural hypotension which is the medical term for your blood pressure dropping when you stand up quickly (often seen in elderly people). Patients with PoTS may also describe a racing heart beat or palpitations. The autonomic nervous system is also involved in gut regulation or housekeeping and helps or instructs our gut to contract in a co-ordinated fashion which pushes food all the way through our gut from the top to the bottom (again you may or may not have heard of the term peristalsis which is what I have just described). A local family practitioner and her neuroradiology consultant husband (who are our wonderful close friends) had told me one night, while literally sitting around the kitchen table, that they had noticed a few patients with PoTS who also had gastrointestinal symptoms like abdominal pain and bloating. They also had seen a few cases of coexisting coeliac disease. Thus our study was born! We aimed to determine the prevalence of self-reported gluten sensitivity and coeliac disease in a cohort of patients with PoTS.

One hundred patients with PoTS were recruited from the syncope clinic. This is a heart or cardiology clinic where we have great colleagues who see patients that faint or feel like they are going to faint but do not have an immediately obvious medical reason to explain their symptoms. So for example, one reason for their syncope may be undiagnosed PoTS. We asked these patients to complete a validated questionnaire which screened for gluten sensitivity. Case notes were reviewed to determine the outcomes of relevant gastrointestinal investigations. Patients on a gluten-free diet ranked on a scale of 0–10 the severity of abdominal pain and PoTS symptoms before and after starting the GFD.

So what did we find? Four of the hundred patients (4%) were actually found to have biopsy-proven coeliac disease. This is a completely new association that has not been reported before. Perhaps more importantly in terms of the number of patients affected, there was a very high self-reporting of gluten sensitivity. The self-reported prevalence of gluten sensitivity was 42%; of these 42 patients 64% (27/42) had placed themselves on a gluten-free diet. Thirty-eight per cent (16/42) of these PoTS gluten sensitive patients had never seen a doctor regarding their gastrointestinal symptoms. Patients felt their abdominal pain had improved since starting a gluten-free diet (the score reduced for most from about 8 out of 10 to 4). The patients, however, did not think their PoTS symptoms had got better. So this is completely hot off the press and we still have so much more work to do but I thought I would share this new data with you. If you have PoTS it may particularly be of great interest. In a nutshell there is a high prevalence of self-reported gluten sensitivity in patients with PoTS. A large proportion of patients have not had their gastrointestinal symptoms investigated in either primary or secondary care. The data also suggests that coeliac disease may be more common in PoTS than the general population, but further studies with appropriately matched controls are required to ascertain the nature of this relationship.

References

1. Isasi C, Colmenero I, Casco F, et al. Fibromyalgia and non-celiac gluten sensitivity: a description with remission of fibromyalgia. *Rheumatol Int* 2014;34(11):1607-12.
2. Rodrigo L, Blanco I, Bobes J, de Serres FJ. Effect of one year of a gluten-free diet on the clinical evolution of irritable bowel syndrome plus fibromyalgia in patients with associated lymphocytic enteritis: a case–control study. *Arthritis Res Ther* 2014;16(4):421.
3. Penny HA, Ferrar M, Atkinson J, Hoggard N, Hadjivassiliou M, West JN, Sanders DS. Is there a relationship between gluten ingestion and postural tachycardia syndrome? *Gut Suppl 1* 2015;64:A144.

CHAPTER 11

The role of gluten in Inflammatory Bowel Disease

I nflammatory Bowel Disease (IBD) is a condition which is reported to affect 400 people out of every 100,000 in the UK (approximately 1 in 250 people) or 1–1.5 million people in the US. IBD is subdivided into four groups. The first I want to mention is Crohn's disease which can affect anywhere between the mouth to the anus. The second group is ulcerative colitis which broadly only occurs within the colon. Now these two forms of IBD account for the vast majority of patients but there are two other forms described. The third is called indeterminate colitis. Indeterminate colitis is the term we use when a patient who has IBD does not fit the criteria exactly for either Crohn's disease or ulcerative colitis. Really what I am saying is that although we have made the diagnosis of IBD we don't know whether it is Crohn's or ulcerative colitis and only time will tell by following up the patient. Finally there is the least common form of IBD which is called microscopic colitis. This is where you have a colon which looks normal at the time of your colonoscopy but the biopsies routinely taken from the normal looking colon when studied under the microscope show inflammation. Thus you can see why it has been termed microscopic colitis. Often the inflammation you see in microscopic colitis is driven by lymphocytes which are the same attack cells that we see in the small bowel that drive coeliac disease. Many patients with IBD have wondered if food plays a role in their symptoms.

In 2007 we published a report trying to understand the relationship between coeliac disease and IBD[1]. We tested more than 300 patients with IBD for coeliac disease using standard coeliac serology. Any individual who was positive had a duodenal biopsy. At the same time we reviewed a group of more than 300 patients with coeliac disease to see if there was anything to suggest IBD. We found that if you had IBD then your risk of having coeliac disease was not really any different to the general population (about 1%). However, if you had coeliac disease then you had ten times the risk of having IBD but the type of IBD you generally had was microscopic colitis, the form of IBD which is driven by lymphocytes. Other investigators have also reported or reproduced these findings and some have even suggested that a gluten-free diet may be an option in the patients with microscopic colitis who have excess lymphocytes in their colon irrespective of whether these patients have coexisting coeliac disease or not.

More recently we have made a further intriguing observation which I would like to share with you. We questioned a group of 145 patients with IBD and found that approximately 28% (40/145) self-reported symptoms related to gluten. Furthermore nine out of these 40 patients were currently on a gluten-free diet. None of these 145 patients had coexisting coeliac disease. So within our group of 145 patients with IBD who were questioned approximately 6% (9/145) were on a gluten-free diet of their own choice even though they did not have coeliac disease. We described that if you have active inflammation with your IBD you were more likely to place yourself on a gluten-free diet.[2]

Finally, in both Crohn's and ulcerative colitis it is possible to develop a tightening or stricture in your bowel as a result of the continuous inflammation. We also observed that if you were a Crohn's patient with a stricture then this was another situation where you favoured a gluten-free approach. How can we explain these findings? Many products which contain gluten not unsurprisingly are bulky or doughy, for example pizza or pasta. Now imagine if you have an inflamed bowel and this makes your bowel either sensitive or in some cases narrowed. Then imagine a ball of pizza dough trying to push its way through? Painful? You bet it would be, so people work out for themselves what makes their symptoms worse and avoid these foods accordingly. This may be nothing more than a physical phenomenon, with no relationship of inflammation being promoted by the gluten contained within the foodstuffs, and just a bulking effect.

An alternative suggestion is being put forward by other researchers who are trying to establish whether gluten causes immune inflammation in the gut of patients with IBD. Investigators have described that a particular antibody Anti-*Saccharomyces cerevisiae* (which I described earlier in Chapter 8) is present in about 65% of Crohn's disease patients. The presence of Anti-*Saccharomyces cerevisiae* may be associated with more aggressive Crohn's disease. A patient who has these antibodies may be more likely to require surgery at some point in the course of their disease. Some studies have shown that the Anti-*Saccharomyces cerevisiae* antibodies disappeared during a gluten-free diet. This phenomenon has been observed particularly when considering children who have IBD.[3]

Another alternative is the recent recognition of Amylase Trypsin Inhibitors (ATIs) which are present in wheat and are now considered to be a significant promoter of immune inflammation. ATIs may be the missing link to scientifically explain what some IBD patients have been noticing and reporting for some time, that their IBD may be improved by avoiding gluten. However, there are still only a limited number of studies describing a relationship between gluten and patients with IBD and this is clearly an area for future research.

References

1. Leeds JS, Hœroldt BS, Sidhu R, Hopper AD, Robinson K, Toulson B, Dixon L, Lobo AJ, McAlindon ME, Sanders DS. Is there an association between coeliac disease and inflammatory bowel disease? A study of relative prevalence with population controls. *Scand J Gastroenterol* 2007;42:1214-20.

2. Aziz I, Branchi F, Pearson K, Priest P, Sanders DS. A study evaluating the bidirectional relationship between inflammatory bowel disease and non-celiac gluten sensitivity. *Inflamm Bowel Dis* 2015;21(4): 847-53.

3. Papp M, Lakatos PL. Serological studies in inflammatory bowel disease: how important are they? *Curr Opin Gastroenterol* 2014; 30(4):359-64.

CHAPTER 12

Fertility and gluten

The relationship between coeliac disease and fertility problems is very well studied and described. Patients with undiagnosed coeliac disease are less likely to be able to conceive than people who have not got coeliac disease. If we go to a subfertility clinic and test for undiagnosed coeliac disease in patients attending for fertility problems, it has been suggested that the level may be as high as 3%.

There are some elegant historical studies looking at men with coeliac disease and showing that their sperm shape, appearance and movement is abnormal. Furthermore female patients with undiagnosed coeliac disease have been reported to have worse pregnancy outcomes. Some studies have suggested intrauterine growth restriction, early or pre-term delivery and low birth weights for their babies. I must balance this by saying there are also studies refuting these birth outcome observations.

The proposed link between coeliac disease and poor birth outcomes is said to be as a result of nutrient deficiencies. For example, low iron, low folate or low vitamin B12 may all be seen in patients with coeliac disease at the time of diagnosis.

Tissue transglutaminase antibodies are (as I have said earlier in Chapter 1) critical both in the development of coeliac disease but also one of the antibodies which we test in order to make the diagnosis of coeliac disease.

So you may think well what do coeliac disease and fertility problems have to do with me if I don't have coeliac disease? Now here is a fact which I have only come to understand recently and is amazing to me. Tissue transglutaminase antibodies have been implicated in the development of the placenta. It may be that tissue transglutaminase antibodies have an inflammatory or immuno-logical role in placental development. Nevertheless if the placenta does not develop appropriately then it is difficult to nourish the foetus. Thus a failure in placental development is related directly to subsequent foetal growth restriction. Recently a group of Dutch investigators performed a population based study looking at 7,046 pregnant women.[1] The study is known as the Generation R study and is an ambitious prospective study aiming to follow through 8,800 mothers with a delivery date from April 2002 to January 2006. The idea is to observe outcomes from foetal life onwards for the babies that are born. The Dutch investigators looked at the presence or absence of tissue transglutaminase anti-bodies in these mothers as well as measuring the actual TTG levels. Patients were then subdivided into three groups. Pregnant women who were negative for the TTG antibody accounted for 6,702 patients out of the 7,046 studied. Patients who had a highly posi-tive TTG antibody (most likely indicating undiagnosed coeliac disease) accounted for 36/7,046. Finally it is already known that TTG antibody is present in some of the general population without having coeliac disease. In this study 308 pregnant women had a TTG antibody which was not as high as the 36 considered to have undiagnosed coeliac disease but viewed as an intermediate level. The investigators then observed that the level of TTG antibody in pregnant women had an inverse relationship with foetal growth. Growth of the foetus was reduced to the greatest extent in patients with the highest level of TTG antibody. Now given everything I have said at the start of this chapter, then this result would not be that surprising. In essence if you have undiagnosed coeliac disease then you are more likely to give birth to a smaller baby. However, what was novel was that the birth weight was also reduced in pregnant women with intermediate levels of TTG antibody and if these patients were HLADQ2 or DQ8 positive then this resulted in a further birth weight reduction. So it would appear that being 'coeliac lite' has consequences beyond perhaps just gastrointestinal symptoms. If I was a pregnant woman or considering pregnancy,

I think this study would make me want to know whether I had a positive TTG antibody blood test at the outset. However, I appreciate that the actual differences in birth weight across the three groups are in the range of 50 to 100 grams so I do not want to be alarming or sensational. It is a fascinating standalone study but I guess we have to watch this space for further developments.

References

1. Kiefte-de Jong JC, Jaddoe VW, Uitterlinden AG, Steegers EA, Willemsen SP, Hofman A, Hooijkaas H, Moll HA. Levels of antibodies against tissue transglutaminase during pregnancy are associated with reduced fetal weight and birth weight. *Gastroenterology* 2013;144(4):726-35.

CHAPTER 13

The interplay between alcohol and gluten, two enemies joining forces!

N ow here is a very speculative theory of mine using a study of my friend Professor Hadjivassiliou to give me some supportive evidence. What do alcohol and coeliac disease both have in common? Coeliac disease opens up the small bowel with its inflammation. It does not matter what you want to call it, leaky gut or increased gut permeability, but it is an absolute consequence of this disease process and even after going on to a gluten-free diet there may still be some increased permeability of the small bowel. Not as much as before but it may still be present. Alcohol has exactly the same effect. These are absolute facts which no medical researcher in our field would dispute. Now here is where it gets interesting. We have previously reported that patients with alcohol related liver disease have a higher presence or prevalence of gliadin antibodies than the general population. When we took a small bowel biopsy in such patients very few actually had coeliac disease. You might well say that you are not surprised at all by my findings. 'Of course,' you would say, 'that is the case because you just told me the small bowel increases in terms of permeability when exposed to alcohol,' so all that has happened is that gluten can cross the small bowel barrier far more readily and thus generate antibodies to gliadin. It could be considered as nothing more than a bystander effect. However, Professor Hadjivassiliou took this observation one step further. He looked at patients with alcohol related ataxia. Ataxia you may recall from Chapter 8 is a condition where the back of your brain or cerebellum is damaged. This means your balance is affected and you may walk unsteadily when even mildly impaired. Ataxia related to alcohol is very common. What our team showed was that in 104 patients with alcohol related ataxia the prevalence of a gliadin antibody was 44% by comparison to the background presence of gliadin antibodies in the general population which was 12%.[1] When we looked at the HLA genetics of the alcohol related ataxia patients, then we found that HLADQ2 or DQ8 was present in 30%. Thus it appears there is some kind of relationship between alcohol and gluten ingestion. We wondered if alcohol related cerebellar degeneration may, in genetically susceptible individuals, induce sensitisation to gluten, or if the genetic susceptibility to gluten enhanced the toxic effect of alcohol on the cerebellum. It remains speculative and we require other investigators to replicate and better our study.

Reference

1. Currie S, Hoggard N, Clark MJ, Sanders DS, Wilkinson ID, Griffiths PD, Hadjivassiliou M. Alcohol induces sensitization to gluten in genetically susceptible individuals: a case–control study. *PLoS One* 2013;8(10):e77638.

CHAPTER 14

The gluten-free diet versus all comers!

Which diet for me?

Obesogenic world

We live in an 'obesogenic'environment and there are calories all around us. The term obesogenic is popularised to reflect that the environment we are currently living in promotes over-eating. It is an environment where high calorie food is readily available. I also think it is in our nature biologically to try and grab those calories when we see them. This comes from our hunter gatherer origins. As hunter gatherers food was a luxury or certainly scarce and there would have been periods of enforced fasting or famine. This meant that when we did have an opportunity to eat we did so with relish as we did not know when such an opportunity would present itself again. This was an attempt to store calories or lay down fat stores which may allow us to survive the next famine. We don't actually want to diet at all as this is not our biological desire. Dieting is really hard. So the way this plays out in modern society is that we are still driven to eat when we have an opportunity, thus in an obesogenic environment (where there is no famine) this results in obesity. This is reflected by society and our ever increasing Body Mass Index (BMI). I don't need to really convince you as all you have to do is look at pictures of Western society at different time points and you can see a progressive change in our collective appearance. Look at pictures of your grandparents or great grandparents dating back to the First or Second World War and the visual differences to modern day society are so apparent. A BMI of over 25 is overweight and 30 is obese and this affects Western populations most of all with approximately 30% overweight and 30% obese. The most significant problem with obesity is within the US but the UK is not far behind as the most overweight European country. A further issue which is fascinating is what I have called relative perception. I have suggested that if we look at historical pictures of our society we will be startled by the relative difference of our ancestors in terms of their BMI by comparison against ourselves. However, if we ask parents of obese children or overweight and obese adults themselves (based strictly on BMI measurements) about what they think of their physical appearance or if they are overweight, up to 75% may consider that this is not the case. This is relative perception: in a nation of people who are overweight or obese, the natural comparison is against people you see on the street or in your daily place of work. If everyone looks similar to you then you may not perceive a problem. This visual mind trick is disastrous from a public health perspective.[1]

Glycaemic index

To understand some aspects of obesity or being overweight it is crucial to understand the glycaemic index. The glycaemic index is based on glucose. If you eat glucose your blood sugar level rises to 100. Everything else we eat in terms of raising blood sugar is compared to that glycaemic index. Why is this important? A high blood sugar is not viewed as a desirable metabolic profile. The clearest problem with persisting high blood sugars that we are all familiar with is diabetes. So the medical profession recommends avoiding or eating in moderation foods with a high glycaemic index.

Which diet for me? Part I

Being obese is associated with an increased mortality for any obese individual by comparison to people who have a normal BMI. Obesity is associated with many other medical complications and thus the medical advice is always with the emphasis on weight loss. This brings us to dieting. However, dieting is not just something which is an issue for overweight or obese people. Dieting is an established part of our modern society. At any given time 20–30% of the population may be on a diet and this may encompass those who are overweight, obese or even normal BMI (for aesthetic reasons). The US spends 20–30 billion dollars on the dieting industry annually. It is a national pastime both in the UK and the US. This has spawned so many different diets. Whichever is the current zeitgeist, you may say. So I thought I would summarise some of what I perceive to be the current or established diets in the following table:

Low Carbohydrate Diet	A self-explanatory diet which involves the reduction or restriction of foodstuffs high in carbohydrates, for example sugar, bread or pasta. Particularly recommended for people suffering with diabetes or obesity.
Low Fat Diet	A self-explanatory diet which involves the reduction or restriction of fat, particularly saturated fats and cholesterol. Recommended for obesity and those at risk of heart disease.
Atkins Diet	A form of low or almost zero carbohydrate intake. Unlimited protein and fat intake, with carbohydrate intake initially restricted to 20 g/day (5–10% of daily calorie intake), mainly as salad greens and other non-starchy vegetables.
Dukan Diet	Again like Atkins a protein based low carbohydrate diet. Low calorie meals and small portions. The foodstuffs are based on a list of 100 with four phases to the diet, attack, cruise, consolidation and stabilisation. Popular for general weight loss.
High Fat (and Protein) Diet	Recently popularised by the release of a book by UK based nutritionist Zana Morris. Careful scrutiny reveals again a key component of the diet to be avoidance of carbohydrates.
Two Day Diet (or 5:2 diet)	Again a protein based low carbohydrate diet. Differs from Atkins and Dukan in the manner of carbohydrate intake. Two consecutive days are spent eating a restricted 500 calories for women and 600 for men. Reported as being easier to undertake as a result of only having a two day restriction.

Paleo Diet	Paleo diet, the diet of our ancestors. Based on what was available in hunter gatherer communities. Chiefly meat, fish, vegetables and fruit, and excluding dairy or cereal products and processed food. Popular with 'lifestylers' and those who believe in a 'free from' approach to food.
Gluten-free Diet	I will say no more. ☺
FODMAP (Fermentable Oligosaccharides, Disaccharides, Monosaccharides, and Polyols)	Popular for Irritable Bowel Syndrome and extensively discussed in Chapter 5.
Mediterranean Diet	A diet with its origins from 1960s to 1970s based on the observations that the Mediterranean population have lower rates of cardiovascular disease. High in legumes, fruits, unrefined cereals, fish and olive oil. Low in meat and saturated fat.
South Beach Diet	A low glycaemic index diet designed for patients with ischaemic heart disease. There is no calorie counting. You eat three meals and two snacks a day and have an associated exercise plan. However, the lean protein, including meat, fish and poultry, can be highly restrictive.

This list is by no means exhaustive but I wanted to show scientific themes being developed as to why the diet works or should work and demonstrate that there are many similarities between these diets.

Zombie statistic

A zombie statistic is a statement of 'fact' which has no apparent substance attached to it. When scrutinised it may not be factually accurate in any way but despite evidence to the contrary the 'zombie statistic' will not die; it keeps coming back to life and being used liberally. Politicians are the best deliverers of zombie statistics. However, in my medical practice a favourite zombie statistic is that 'a gluten-free diet will help me lose weight'. There is no substance to this claim. There are two medical reasons which are cited for this statement. The first is that whole wheat bread has a high glycaemic index of greater than 70. This fact is always described in comparison to other foodstuffs (which we may perceive as bad for us or as treats), for example peanut M&Ms have a glycaemic index of more than 30 and Snickers approximately greater than 50. So at face value bread looks like it is worse for you based on the glycaemic index. When you actually start looking at the glycaemic index of many foodstuffs and look beyond the simple comparison I have provided, you realise that there are many foodstuffs which we accept as part of our healthy balanced diet that also have a high glycaemic index. For example, Bran Flakes and Corn Flakes both have a glycaemic index of more than 70. So glycaemic index although important is not the whole story. The second medical reason is that laboratory based rodent studies have suggested that gluten has an opiate-like effect. In *Wheat Belly* (written by Dr William Davis) there is a section termed 'bread is my crack'. In Chapter 8 when I discussed the brain–gut axis I mentioned gluten opioids which are able to cross the blood–brain barrier. So the suggestion here is that these gluten opioids make you want to eat more gluten and so you enter a vicious circle which ultimately ends in obesity. There is very little published scientific evidence to support this statement. There is absolutely no doubt, however, that reducing gluten can be a surrogate way of reducing carbohydrate intake. If you remove pizza, pasta and bread from your diet and this accounts for a significant portion of your daily calories, then of course you will lose weight.

Which diet for me? Part II

So here is what it comes down to as I see it. The average caloric intake for men is 2,500 calories per day and 2,000 for women. Fat provides 9 calories per gram while carbohydrates and protein each provide 4 calories per gram. In a recent study 19 obese patients agreed to cut their calories from initially 2,700 calories per day (at the start of the study) to 1,800 calories by reducing either carbohydrates or fat. What happened was that after six days on each diet, those reducing fat intake lost an average 463g of body fat – 80% more than those cutting down on carbohydrates, whose average loss was 245g.[2]

Clearly based on calories per gram the more fat you avoid the greater the calorie loss because it is 9 calories per gram. However, the investigators very sensibly concluded that dieting is really about whatever works for you. At the end of the day the maths add up: if you eat a certain amount of calories you gain or lose weight accordingly. Any diet is merely a tool to aid you should you require it. A healthy balanced diet is by far and away the optimal approach and many of the diets I have outlined may be of value in the short term reduction of weight but may not allow you to sustain the weight loss. Thus adopting an overall approach to healthy eating both in terms of calories and nutrition may be of greater benefit. It is just not that easy in an obesogenic environment; believe me, I know, and I am no different to anyone else!

What is a gluten-free diet?

In medicine I like considering options for patients in a methodical way. It is what I and others call risks, benefits, alternatives and nothing. In this chapter we have discussed the variety of diets that are available. I would describe this as 'alternatives'. However, if you are considering a gluten-free diet for symptoms, non-coeliac gluten sensitivity or coeliac disease then this next section will help you decide.

A gluten-free diet has been the accepted treatment for coeliac disease since the 1950s after the historical work of Dr Dicke (whom I mentioned in Chapter 1, who made the seminal observations regarding a gluten-free diet). This means we have almost 70 years' experience of this diet, which far outstrips any of the dietary options we have discussed in this chapter.

There are three elements to a gluten-free diet. Eating naturally gluten-free food such as corn, rice or potatoes; I am just giving some examples and this is by no means exhaustive. If you are seeking advice about a gluten-free diet because you have been diagnosed with coeliac disease or considering the diet for other reasons, I would strongly recommend looking at the Coeliac UK website irrespective of where you live in the world (www.coeliac.

org.uk/). There are other websites for different countries and many of them are excellent. There are also many uncontrolled websites which are sources of misinformation! The reason I recommend the Coeliac UK website is because Coeliac UK are the oldest and largest charity founded in 1968 to support patients. They want to support all people who have symptoms related to eating gluten, both coeliac patients and those with non-coeliac gluten sensitivity. It is their crossed grain sign which is internationally used to designate safety for gluten-free products. I am honoured to currently chair their Health Advisory Council and thus I have a unique knowledge of their website and what the brilliant and passionate staff of Coeliac UK has to offer patients in terms of support. I would start there but then spread your wings cautiously across the internet. Most importantly the key message of this chapter:

> **Rule number 7:**
>
> A dietitian is the cornerstone of management for patients who require a gluten-free diet.

So I have mentioned naturally occurring gluten-free foods but the other two elements to a gluten-free diet are avoidance of gluten-containing processed food, for example pasta, pizza, bread, cakes and of course food products with barley and rye. The list is endless. Finally there is the positive selection of commercial food which has been manufactured to the internationally accepted gluten-free standards.

In 2008 the Codex Alimentarius Commission of the World Health Organisation defined and agreed that food which contains 20 ppm (parts per million) of gluten was the standard for gluten-free products. What does this mean? This means 1 kilogram of food X will contain no more than 20 milligrams of gluten. The 20 parts per million comes from this: 1kg is 1,000 grams and 1 gram is 1,000 milligrams. Thus 1 kilogram contains 1,000,000 milligrams (1 million). So 20 milligrams in 1 million milligrams is 20 parts per million. Sorry if that was hard work but if you are considering a gluten-free diet then I think it is worth understanding this phrase of 20 ppm as it comes up all the time. In the USA the Food and Drug Administration (FDA) have also agreed and approved this standard.[3]

The prospect of a gluten-free diet can be daunting. We (the medical profession) have certainly learnt from patients with coeliac disease that the key to success in terms of being able to cope with the gluten-free diet is education. Knowledge is power and this enables you to understand the complexities of the diet. Patients with coeliac disease have reported that dietetic support, patient charities and local networks make it easier to stick to the diet and make them feel less isolated or vulnerable.

Controversies of a gluten-free diet

Although we have set the standard as 20 ppm for what is accepted as gluten-free there are some coeliac patients who will even respond adversely to this level of exposure to gluten. The research done on gluten thresholds is interesting as it reveals that doctors can set the 'rules' but humans don't follow them! When small amounts of gluten are placed directly into the small bowel (within the duodenum) of people with coeliac disease (who agreed to take part in this research and were stable on a gluten-free diet) there was individual variation for the amount of gluten which was required before they developed changes on biopsy. A double blind placebo study which challenged patients with gluten showed that at a level of 10mg of gluten per day over three months there were few changes on biopsy but for the group given 50 mg per day over three months this resulted in the biopsy showing inflammation. So it does seem sensible to set the standard at 20 parts per million but there will be individuals who are super sensitive and their immune system will respond even on the standard gluten-free diet. I then suggest trying a wheat-free gluten-free diet or a naturally gluten-free diet.

Oats are nutritionally rich alternative grains that have been shown to lower blood sugar, reduce lipids (of the unwanted type) and increase our dietary fibre. However, there are two controversies, the first being that of cross contamination. Cross contamination is the fact that no legislation exists to separate the processing of gluten-containing cereals (wheat, barley and rye) from oats. An American and Canadian based study tested 134 oat grain products and revealed that 109 were cross contaminated. So this report suggests more than 80% contamination (109/134) which can only be avoided by looking for the crossed grain sign. This means on a practical level that although I encourage patients to consume oats I recommend that they stick to products which describe themselves as gluten-free oats and have the crossed grain sign. The second controversy is that for a small percentage of patients their immune system recognises the oats incorrectly. Oats is seen as a 'gluten like' protein and the outcome is that those people have an adverse immune response to oats. This I term molecular mimicry, in other words for their bad luck oats has been placed in the same camp as gluten-containing cereals. There is no real way around this other than oats avoidance but it is uncommon, perhaps 1–5% of patients with coeliac disease, and for the non-coeliac gluten sensitive individual this may be even less and not something which the patients have generally reported to me.

The nutritional content of a gluten-free diet is the source of both controversy and sometimes misinformation. International studies have undertaken nutritional assessments of coeliac patients who are either newly diagnosed or have been on a gluten-free diet for some time. Within this specific coeliac patient cohort it has been reported in some studies that the intake of both vitamins and minerals is inadequate. This does not equate to the inadequacy of the gluten-free diet as the issue is multifactorial. Patients with newly diagnosed coeliac disease or who are not adhering to the gluten-free diet will not absorb nutrients optimally so this is an alternative reason for this problem. Individual patients' eating habits may also explain nutritional inadequacies. Society as a whole may be neglectful of eating a balanced and nutritionally adequate diet.

There have been reports that a gluten-free diet is high in simple sugars, saturated fat and low in fibre and that gluten-free manufactured foods have a high glycaemic index. However, there are just as many dietary assessments of the gluten-free diet which document that this is not the case.

Another strand of evidence which is pointed to is that individuals with newly diagnosed coeliac disease gain weight on a gluten-free diet. If you have malabsorption then it is hardly surprising that when you start a gluten-free diet the villi grow back and you end up absorbing nutrients, calories and thus gain weight. This does not mean the gluten-free diet is the culprit for weight gain. Furthermore in this 'obesogenic' environment many investigators have reported that the majority of adult coeliac patients at the time of diagnosis have a normal Body Mass Index or can even be overweight or obese with a raised BMI. This simply reflects society, and comes back to what I said earlier which is that a BMI of over 25 is overweight and 30 is obese, and Western populations have the most significant problem, with obesity within the US leading the way and the UK not far behind as the most overweight European country.

A recent study which is worthy of mention looks at something called the metabolic syndrome.[4] The metabolic syndrome is defined as risk factors for Type II diabetes and cardiovascular disease (abdominal obesity, high blood pressure, high levels of the wrong lipids and problems with glucose regulation). In this study of 98 patients with coeliac disease, two of the 98 had metabolic syndrome at the time of diagnosis and 12 months after a gluten-free diet this number rose to 29/98. So a change from 2% to 30%, but currently metabolic syndrome is estimated to affect up to 25% of the world's total population and this figure is even higher in our high socio-economic countries. All that has really happened is that individuals with undiagnosed coeliac disease who have previously been unable to absorb all the calories that they eat are placed on a gluten-free diet and for the first time absorb those calories. Twelve months down the line they essentially reflect the same picture metabolically as the rest of society. They have caught up! This should not happen if such patients are given and adhere to appropriate nutritional advice. Back to rule number seven. A dietitian is the cornerstone of management for patients who require a gluten-free diet.

This data should not be misrepresented as evidence that either a gluten-free diet is 'bad for you' or a means of 'keeping the pounds off'.

Finally I would say this: we have known for many years that a gluten-free diet improves quality of life for the majority of patients with coeliac disease and now we see similar evidence emerging from patients with non-coeliac gluten sensitivity.[5]

References

1. Jeffery AN, Voss LD, Metcalf BS, Alba S, Wilkin TJ. Parents' awareness of overweight in themselves and their children: cross sectional study within a cohort (EarlyBird 21). *BMJ* 2005;330(7481):23-4.

2. Hall KD, Bemis T, Brychta R, Chen KY, Courville A, Crayner EJ, Goodwin S, Guo J, Howard L, Knuth ND, Miller BV 3rd, Prado CM, Siervo M, Skarulis MC, Walter M, Walter PJ, Yannai L. Calorie for Calorie, Dietary Fat Restriction Results in More Body Fat Loss than Carbohydrate Restriction in People with Obesity. *Cell Metab* 2015; 22(3):427-36.

3. Ciacci C, Ciclitira P, Hadjivassiliou M, Kaukinen K, Ludvigsson JF, McGough N, Sanders DS, Woodward J, Leonard JN, Swift GL. The gluten-free diet and its current application in coeliac disease and dermatitis herpetiformis. *United European Gastroenterol J* 2015; 3(2):121-35.

4. Tortora R, Capone P, De Stefano G, Imperatore N, Gerbino N, Donetto S, Monaco V, Caporaso N, Rispo A. Metabolic syndrome in patients with coeliac disease on a gluten-free diet. *Aliment Pharmacol Ther* 2015;41(4):352-9.

5. Coburn JA, Vande Voort JL, Lahr BD, Van Dyke CT, Kroning CM, Wu TT, Gandhi MJ, Murray JA. Human leukocyte antigen genetics and clinical features of self-treated patients on a gluten-free diet. *J Clin Gastroenterol* 2013;47(10):828-33.

CHAPTER 15

Gluten took my pet!

Gluten took my pet! Off the wall perhaps but I want to walk you through this chapter and the evidence because what I think it demonstrates is that we are not the only mammals struggling with gluten. This is important because it may provide supporting evidence for my assertion in Chapter 1 that wheat is on the rise and with this comes gluten related disorders.

Back in in 1991 the department of Veterinary Pathology in Liverpool published the first of a series of fascinating reports. The authors initially demonstrated that Irish Setter dogs had increased intestinal permeability (leaky gut) on small bowel biopsies. They then designed a really elegant series of studies. They took Irish Setter dogs that were reared 'from the gun' on a wheat-containing diet and showed that small bowel biopsies revealed partial villus atrophy or a slightly flat bowel but also with intraepithelial lymphocyte infiltration (those IELs again!), and increased intestinal permeability. By comparison they also investigated family members of the affected Irish Setter (littermates) who were reared exclusively on a wheat-free or cereal-free diet.

When they gave the affected Irish Setters a gluten-free diet this resulted in an improvement of the biopsy findings from the small bowel, and the small bowel permeability also improved. After these affected dogs had been on a gluten-free diet for some time they were then reintroduced to gluten which resulted in a relapse and a reoccurrence of the pathological changes I described earlier in their small bowel. In contrast, littermates reared exclusively on a cereal-free diet showed minimal changes when challenged with gluten, apart from intraepithelial lymphocyte infiltration at a low level in some instances. This was the first report of gluten sensitive enteropathy (or dog equivalent of coeliac disease) in Irish Setters. The clinical message to vets and owners alike was to consider exclusion of dietary wheat and/or cereals from birth in order to try and avoid the development of this disease in the future. So here is the first non-human model of coeliac disease which is clearly demonstrated and undisputed.[1]

Research is always fascinating and through research you often meet amazing people with curious questioning minds. This brings me to Mark Lowrie. Mark Lowrie is a Cambridge and Glasgow University trained vet whom I have not met but email corresponded and collaborated with. He and his colleagues work in Hertfordshire and his inquisitive mind led him to making a unique observation which I would like to tell you about. Canine Epileptoid Cramping Syndrome (CECS) is a movement disorder which affects Border Terriers. The terriers do not have control of these movements; there are features which are neurologically similar to what my friend Professor Hadjivassiliou has described in humans (in Chapter 8). I know this also because I have seen the videos of these animals suffering with this disorder and the uncontrolled movements appear very similar to what I have seen over the years in adults through working alongside Professor Hadjivassiliou. Episodes may be seen in Border Terriers as young as six weeks old but can even present as late as seven years old. The involuntary movements may be so severe that when they occur the dog cannot move its limbs. These episodes may last from minutes to hours occurring recurrently during a single 'bout' over the course of a day. In between the dog may be well for months or years. It is thought that stress or excitement might be an initiator in these events. An important feature may be gastrointestinal symptoms which occur in tandem with the neurological symptoms. Mark and his colleagues took six affected Border Terriers and checked them for tissue transglutaminase antibodies and antigliadin antibodies when they first presented. Either tissue transglutaminase antibodies or antigliadin antibodies or both were elevated in all six dogs. These dogs were then placed on a gluten-free diet. The antibody panel was then repeated at specific time points after commencing a gluten-free diet as a non-invasive way of checking adherence. After nine months five out of the six dogs showed improvement not only on their blood tests but also critically a clinical reduction in the number of episodes that these dogs suffered with. There was one dog that had persisting symptoms and positive antibodies and this particular dog was found to be scavenging horse manure which results in the inadvertent consumption of gluten. Once this was rectified this Border Terrier also responded.[2] This unique report is of course what we call a case series. In other words it is not a randomised study of the effects of a gluten-free diet on Border Terriers affected by CECS, but I believe this is a seminal observation and the beginning of establishing this link between gluten and neurological disturbances in Border Terriers. It was concluded in the study that CECS may in the future be described as a gluten sensitive movement disorder.

I entitled this chapter 'Gluten took my pet!' not to be flippant or frivolous but to catch your eye. If you were the owner of either Irish Setters or Border Terriers I think you would be very grateful for the work done by these inquisitive research orientated vets. Their observations will have improved the wellbeing of these dogs. For me I would like to try and suggest that this is objective proof of gluten still being biologically 'new' to either humans or, in this case, dogs and demonstrating how it provokes our immune system resulting in a deleterious effect.

References

1. Hall EJ, Batt RM. Dietary modulation of gluten sensitivity in a naturally occurring enteropathy of Irish setter dogs. *Gut* 1992;33(2): 198-205.
2. Lowrie M, Garden O, Hadjivassiliou M, Harvey RJ, Sanders DS, Powell R, Garosi L. Canine Epileptoid Cramping Syndrome: Does Gluten play a role? *Journal of Veterinary Internal Medicine* 2015; 29:1564-8.

Conclusion

I would like to summarise my perspective. It has also been a learning experience for me to have to commit my view to paper so extensively. Gluten is ubiquitous and sneaks in everywhere unbeknown to us, most likely in ever increasing quantities. Coeliac disease is common and rising and we are seeing an increasing trend of other gluten related disorders. The HLA genetic association must always be present for coeliac disease to occur and we have seen in the reported literature that an HLADQ2 or DQ8 associated 'coeliac lite' patient may also benefit from a gluten-free diet if symptomatic. The emerging entity of non-coeliac gluten sensitivity requires so much more international scientific study (perhaps the rest of my career!).

If you do have symptoms that you think may be related to gluten then it is essential that you make no changes to your diet. Seek medical advice first and foremost and be persuasive! It is critical to get this right for yourself at the outset. Knowing whether or not you have coeliac disease or non-coeliac gluten sensitivity has implications for you and your family and affects the rest of your life.

Eating is not just an act of nutritional requirements. Eating is central to our lives and has great social importance. Any problems with eating gluten can have a very negative impact on your food related quality of life. I have previously shown the significant negative impact that coeliac disease has on affected individuals with particular regard to daily social restrictions. I want to introduce you to a new term: 'Orthorexia nervosa'. This condition is not currently recognised as a clinical diagnosis but many people struggle with symptoms related to eating food so I felt it important to mention and define this condition. Orthorexia nervosa is said to describe individuals who have an 'unhealthy obsession' with otherwise healthy eating. Orthorexia nervosa is described as a 'fixation on righteous eating'. It is considered that this starts out as an innocent attempt to eat more healthily, but orthorexics may become fixated on food quality and purity. This can then progress to other features: 'what and how much to eat', and how to deal with 'slip-ups'. Ultimately this obsession can become a central facet of their lifestyle or personality. I would not wish this problem on anyone and thus for me knowledge of gluten and your relationship with gluten is power to you. There is a lot of sensationalism and hype surrounding that devil gluten! I would like to think that this book will help to advise you and empower you both in terms of understanding the evidence and providing guidance about how best to look after yourself.

I keep wondering if gluten is a public health problem. We all accept that we should try and achieve our five portions (or even seven!) of fruit and vegetables per day and I wonder if there is a similar story to be told for gluten. Should we all ensure we only have five grams or ten grams per day? Should it just be those who have identified problems when they eat gluten (as long as they have been through the appropriate diagnostic pathways)? Or should it be preventative in order to avoid developing antibodies? It is difficult to say, and time (and further research) will tell, but certainly as we have discovered in the course of these chapters commercial gluten usage is unregulated and appears to have many, many unexplained effects and associations.

Medical practice is a very conservative beast and rightly so because this provides a safety net for patients. Doctors behave within the conservative boundaries of medicine. '*Primum non nocere*', first do no harm, an excellent tenet for all doctors. However, the one fly in this ointment is the slow pace for new developments or acceptance of a change in our medically taught practices. Thomas Samuel Kuhn (1922–1996) was an American physicist, historian, and philosopher of science. He introduced a term we are all familiar with in our contemporary society. The concept of a paradigm shift was first described in his book *The Structure of Scientific Revolutions* (published in 1962). One aspect of the Kuhnian model which is at odds with modern medicine is that opposing theories can coexist. In medicine we may view this with great suspicion as we broadly like a mathematical approach to patients, 2 + 2 = 4. There can be no other answers or diagnosis. But human beings and their bodies don't always listen to our logical science. As doctors we have to be very careful not to convert our scientific knowledge into ideology.

For you, reading this book out of interest, I hope I have shared the unbiased evidence with you and now you will make your own mind up.

Rule number 8 of Gluten Attack:

Gluten is not the devil but there is much hype and sensationalism that may drive our concerns.

Rule number 9 of Gluten Attack:

Gluten may be an emerging public health problem.

Rule number 10 of Gluten Attack:

Ultimately the evidence will represent itself and you will determine and formulate your own view.

Rules of Gluten Attack

Rule number 1 of Gluten Attack: If you have symptoms when you eat gluten please please go and see a doctor. Do not place yourself on a gluten-free diet no matter how fed up you may be (even with doctors!). Try to clarify the diagnosis medically once and for all.

Rule number 2 of Gluten Attack: There is no need for everyone to be on a gluten-free diet and if it is a lifestyle choice that you have made then currently it is without proof.

Rule number 3 of Gluten Attack: It is okay for you to ask your doctor if you can be tested for coeliac disease.

Rule number 4 of Gluten Attack: *Primum non nocere*, first do no harm to yourself and if you are unhappy with the medical advice you have been given seek a second opinion.

Rule number 5 of Gluten Attack: The absence of evidence should not be used as proof of no effect.

Rule number 6 of Gluten Attack: Understanding the differences between wheat allergy, coeliac disease and food intolerance may help you manage your symptoms.

Rule number 7 of Gluten Attack: If you have unexplained neurological symptoms then knowing whether you have positive gluten related antibodies or coeliac disease is important.

Rule number 8 of Gluten Attack: Gluten is not the devil but there is much hype and sensationalism that may drive our concerns.

Rule number 9 of Gluten Attack: Gluten may be an emerging public health problem.

Rule number 10 of Gluten Attack: Ultimately the evidence will represent itself and you will determine and formulate your own view.

Epilogue

An outdoor garden trampoline has very specific physical properties. I have a colleague, a general practitioner from Kent, UK, who has a brilliant spontaneous soap box rant about the dangers of a trampoline. I bought one anyway. It actually requires the heaviest person to be in the middle to get the best elevation for the others. In a nutshell you need a heavy adult in the centre of the trampoline (jumping up and down in a steady rhythm) so that all the kids get maximum bounce around the peripheries. (This is entirely contrary to the set of instructions that accompany the trampoline!) The first time we worked this out we were singing 'Wild Thing' (The Troggs, 1966) as we bounced higher and higher giggling wildly at the thrill of it. Based on that experience the kids coined the descriptive phrase for me of 'wild fat'. My son's friend Charlie, when asked what type of animal he thought I would be, helpfully volunteered that 'Dave is a pot bellied pig'. Thus was born the descriptive term for me of wild fat pot bellied pig! Kids are so cruel! Much truth said in jest. Nevertheless the kids are the joy of my little world.

Dan, our son, drew a picture of a sleek elegant cheetah eating a pot bellied pig. The cheetah he said is his mum. This tells you something about the dynamics in our household.

I am sitting at my kitchen table facing out onto our garden, typing. This book has been five years in the making. The kids come past me. We have two children, an eight year old boy and an eleven year old girl. They are both vibrant and very quick witted. They are their mother's children. Their friend Becky chips in, 'What's he doing?' 'My dad's writing a book,' replies Samira (AKA Simmy).

'He is so boring,' she follows through. 'What's it about?' asks Becky. 'It's all about the gluten,' Simmy replies. In one sentence she summarises 20 years of work ...

'C'mmon, wild fat pot bellied pig,' Dan shouts, 'get on the trampoline.' Kids are a great leveller. It is important not to take oneself too seriously.

People are interesting: they often have a story to tell which bears relevance to all of us. Medicine is the same. If we listen to our patients they can show us new frontiers of medicine, if we just open our minds and listen. Medicine in my opinion is neither a science nor an art; it is an amazing blend of both. This is because, as I said earlier, people (our patients) do not fit perfectly into boxes; we are simply not mathematical models. Science tries to apply this approach for the benefit of society (and that is broadly good) but every now and then an individual person does not fit our scientific rationale. This is the 'art' of medicine, knowing the difference. I am not sure if I know the difference. I am certainly not a patch on my father or Professor Bardhan but I am trying my best. Of course you are the judge of this. I started this book by suggesting that I would like to share the unbiased evidence with you and let you make your own mind up. I hope sincerely that I have achieved this.

Now for me, duty calls on the trampoline and, for you in the following part of this book, something much lighter and completely different.

Thank you for reading.

Recipes

BERRY PANCAKES

Serves 4

Ingredients

125g gluten-free flour
½ tsp ground cinnamon
1 tsp gluten-free baking powder
1 egg
175ml milk
25g unsalted butter, melted
50g blueberries
50g raspberries
25g strawberries, hulled and halved
1 tbsp olive oil
maple syrup to serve (optional)

Method

1. In a large bowl mix together the flour, cinnamon and baking powder.
2. Whisk together the egg and milk and then whisk into the dry ingredients until smooth – the mixture should be the consistency of thick double cream.
3. Stir in the melted butter and half of the berries.

4. Heat the oil in a frying pan over a medium heat, then spoon tablespoons of the batter into the pan. Cook for 2–3 minutes until golden underneath and then flip over and cook for a further 2–3 minutes.
5. Repeat with the remaining batter.
6. Serve with the remaining berries and a drizzle of maple syrup if wished.

BREAKFAST SMOOTHIE BOWL

Serves 4

Ingredients

100g raspberries
100g blackberries
2 small bananas, peeled and sliced
700ml milk
2 tbsp natural yoghurt
4 tbsp muesli
1 tbsp pumpkin seeds
4 tbsp blueberries

Method

1. Place the raspberries, blackberries, 1 sliced banana, milk, yoghurt and half the muesli in a blender and blend until smooth. Add a little more milk if too thick to pour.
2. Pour into four bowls and top with the remaining ingredients to serve.

EGGS FLORENTINE

Serves 4

Ingredients

4 tbsp white wine vinegar
6 peppercorns
sprig of tarragon
4 egg yolks
225g butter
1 tbsp lemon juice
seasoning
4 eggs
300g spinach leaves
2 avocado, peeled, destoned and sliced

Method

1. Place the vinegar in a small pan with the peppercorns and tarragon. Reduce over a high heat until only 2 tbsp remain. Strain.
2. In a food processor or blender, blend together the egg yolks and vinegar reduction.
3. Gently melt the butter in another small pan, letting the solids fall to the bottom of the pan.
4. With the food processor running, slowly pour the melted butter into the egg yolks. The sauce will start to thicken. Stop when only the butter solids are left.
5. Season with lemon juice and seasoning to taste, adding a little water to loosen if needed. Keep warm.
6. Meanwhile, poach the eggs in a simmering frying pan of water and pour boiling water over the spinach in a colander.
7. Arrange the slices of avocado on four plates, top with the spinach and then 1 egg, and pour over the hollandaise sauce to serve.

GRUYERE AND PANCETTA HASHBROWNS, WITH POACHED EGGS

Serves 4

Ingredients

4 slices pancetta
5 eggs
4 medium potatoes, peeled and grated
100g Gruyere cheese, grated
1 small onion, peeled and finely sliced
seasoning
2 tbsp olive oil
2 tbsp chopped chives to serve

Method

1. Grill the slices of pancetta for 2–3 minutes on each side, until nearly crisp. Roughly chop.
2. Beat 1 egg in a large bowl and mix together with the pancetta, grated potato, cheese, onion and seasoning.
3. Heat the oil in a large frying pan and add spoonfuls of the potato mixture and then flatten into patties about 1cm thick. Cook for 2–3 minutes on each side, until crisp and golden (you may need to do this in batches, so keep warm while cooking remaining mixture).
4. Meanwhile poach remaining eggs in a frying pan of simmering water.
5. Serve the hashbrowns topped with a poached egg and scattering of chives.

SWEET POTATO AND GOAT'S CHEESE FRITTATA

Serves 4

Ingredients

350g sweet potato, peeled and chopped
2 tbsp olive oil
1 red onion, peeled and chopped
1 red pepper, deseeded and sliced
125g fresh or frozen peas
7 eggs
1 tbsp chopped mint
1 tbsp snipped chives
75g goat's cheese
seasoning

Method

1. Cook the sweet potato in a pan of boiling water for 8 minutes, until just tender. Drain.
2. Heat half the olive oil in a frying pan and cook the onion with the sweet potato and red pepper slices for 5–6 minutes. Add the peas and cook for one minute more.
3. Beat the eggs in a large bowl, pour in the vegetables and mix well. Season and stir in the herbs.
4. Heat the remaining oil in the same frying pan and pour the egg and vegetables back into the pan. Cook over a low heat for 15–18 minutes, until the bottom of the fritatta is golden (you can check this using a spatula to pull a little away from the side of the pan).
5. Preheat the grill to hot.
6. Crumble over the goat's cheese and place the pan under the grill for 6–8 minutes, until the cheese is melted and the fritatta is golden.
7. Leave the fritatta to stand for a minute then run a knife around the edge of the pan, place a plate or board on top and turn over to remove from the pan.
8. Cut into wedges to serve.

CHEESE & LEEK MACARONI

Serves 4

Ingredients

350g gluten-free macaroni
75g butter
1 leek, trimmed and finely sliced
50g gluten-free flour
1 tsp English mustard powder
700ml milk
175g mature Cheddar cheese, grated
50g Parmesan, grated
seasoning
crisp green salad to serve

Method

1. Preheat the oven to 190°C (375°F) Gas mark 5.
2. Cook the macaroni according to the pack instructions, until al dente (still has a little 'bite').
3. Meanwhile, melt the butter in a pan and sauté the sliced leeks for 6–8 minutes, until softened.
4. Stir the flour and mustard powder into the leeks and cook, stirring, for 1 minute.
5. Gradually add the milk, a little at a time, stirring constantly, until thickened. Bring to a simmer and cook for 2 minutes before stirring in all but 2 tbsp of the Cheddar cheese. Season.
6. Drain the macaroni and pour into the cheese and leek sauce – mix thoroughly to coat all of the pasta with sauce.
7. Pour into an ovenproof dish and sprinkle over the remaining cheeses. Bake in the preheated oven for 15–20 minutes, until bubbling and golden.
8. Serve with crisp green salad.

CHICKEN TACOS WITH RED PEPPER SALSA

Serves 4

Ingredients

2 red peppers, deseeded and diced
4 spring onions, trimmed and sliced
¼ cucumber, diced
handful parsley, chopped
juice of ½ lemon
1 tbsp extra virgin olive oil
1 tbsp olive oil
4 chicken breasts, cut into thin strips
1 red onion, peeled and thinly sliced
½ tsp paprika
2 garlic cloves, crushed
1 red chilli, deseeded and finely chopped
4 tomatoes, chopped
2 little gem lettuces, shredded
8 taco shells

Method

1. To make the salsa, mix together the diced peppers, spring onions and cucumber with the parsley, lemon juice and extra virgin olive oil. Leave to stand at room temperature.
2. Heat the oil in a frying pan or wok and cook the chicken to brown all over.
3. Add the onion and cook for 2–3 minutes before sprinkling in the paprika, garlic and chilli. Cook for 1 minute.
4. Stir in the tomatoes and cook for a further minute.
5. Divide the shredded lettuce between the taco shells and then top with the chicken and finally a dollop of salsa.

CURRIED BUTTERNUT SOUP

Serves 4

Ingredients

1 tbsp olive oil
1 tsp mustard seeds
1 tsp cumin seeds
1 onion, peeled and chopped
1 garlic clove, peeled and chopped
500g butternut squash, chopped
2 carrots, peeled and chopped
2 tsp curry powder
100g red lentils
700ml vegetable stock
1 x 400g can coconut milk
handful coriander leaves to serve

Method

1. Heat the olive oil in a pan, add the mustard and cumin seeds and cook until they start to 'pop'.
2. Add the onion and garlic and sauté for 3–4 minutes.
3. Add the butternut and carrot and cook for another 3–4 minutes before stirring in the curry powder and red lentils.
4. Pour in the stock and coconut milk, bring to a simmer and cook for 15–18 minutes, until the vegetables are tender.
5. Using a hand blender or food processor, blend until smooth.
6. Serve sprinkled with coriander leaves.

FRESH TUNA SALAD NICOISE

Serves 4

Ingredients

3 tbsp extra virgin olive oil
juice of 1 lemon
2 tsp honey
2 tsp Dijon mustard
1 tbsp snipped chives
seasoning
1 tbsp olive oil
4 tuna steaks
8 new potatoes, halved
120g green beans, trimmed
4 eggs
3 little gem lettuces, leaves separated
1 small red onion, peeled and thinly sliced
16 pitted black olives
8 cherry tomatoes, halved
6 anchovy fillets, cut lengthways into thin strips
small handful basil leaves, roughly torn

Method

1. To make the dressing, whisk together the extra virgin olive oil, lemon juice, honey, mustard, chives and seasoning.
2. Heat the olive oil in a griddle or frying pan and cook the tuna steaks for 4–5 minutes on each side, depending on how rare you like your tuna. Remove from the heat and leave to rest.
3. Cook the new potatoes in a small pan of boiling water for 12–15 minutes, adding the beans for the last 3 minutes of cooking. Drain and refresh the vegetables under cold running water.

4. Softly boil the eggs then place in a bowl of cold water before shelling.
5. Place the lettuce leaves on a platter and scatter over the potatoes and green beans.
6. Halve the eggs and add these to the platter.
7. Break the tuna into chunks and place on the platter with the remaining ingredients.
8. Drizzle with the dressing to serve.

HARISSA PRAWN SKEWERS WITH AVOCADO SALAD

Serves 4

Ingredients

500g king prawns
2 tsp harissa paste
4 tbsp olive oil
2 tsp soy sauce
juice of 1½ lemons
1 tsp sesame seeds, toasted
2 garlic cloves, crushed
1 cos lettuce, shredded
12 cherry tomatoes, halved
4 radishes, trimmed and finely sliced
4 spring onions, trimmed and finely sliced
¼ cucumber, sliced
2 avocado, peeled, destoned and sliced
1 tsp honey
1 tsp Dijon mustard
2 tbsp snipped chives

Method

1. Place the prawns in a non-metallic bowl.
2. Whisk together the harissa paste, 1 tbsp olive oil, soy sauce, juice of ½ lemon and sesame seeds. Pour over the prawns and leave to marinate. Soak 8 bamboo skewers in water to prevent them from burning during cooking.
3. Meanwhile, toss together the lettuce, cherry tomatoes, radishes, spring onions, cucumber and avocado.
4. Whisk together the remaining olive oil, lemon juice, honey and mustard.
5. Heat a griddle or grill to hot.
6. Thread the prawns onto the soaked skewers and cook on the griddle or under the grill for 4–5 minute on each side, until they turn pink and are cooked through.
7. Serve the prawn skewers on a bed of salad with the dressing drizzled over the top.

INDIVIDUAL PROSCIUTTO AND ASPARAGUS QUICHES

Makes 12

Ingredients

1 tbsp olive oil
1 onion, peeled and diced
12 slices prosciutto, chopped
125g asparagus tips, trimmed and halved
50g frozen peas
8 eggs
50ml milk
seasoning
80g Parmesan, grated

Method

1. Preheat the oven to 180°C (350°F) Gas mark 4. Lightly grease a 12-hole muffin tin (you can line with paper cases if liked).
2. Heat the oil in a frying pan and sauté the onion for 4–5 minutes, until starting to soften.
3. Add the prosciutto and cook for a further minute before adding the asparagus and peas and cooking for another 2–3 minutes.
4. In a large bowl, beat together the eggs, milk, seasoning, and half of the grated Parmesan.
5. Pour the cooked vegetables into the egg mixture and mix together well.
6. Spoon into the prepared muffin tin and sprinkle over the remaining cheese.
7. Bake for 18–20 minutes, until set and golden.
8. Allow to cool a little before removing from the tin. Serve warm or cold.

JEWELLED LENTILS WITH GRIDDLED HALLOUMI

Serves 4

Ingredients

4 tbsp olive oil
1 red onion, peeled and sliced
1 yellow pepper, deseeded and diced
1 garlic clove, peeled and sliced
1 x 410g can green lentils, drained and rinsed
1 tbsp balsamic vinegar
1 tsp wholegrain mustard
1 tsp honey
seeds from 1 pomegranate
2 tbsp walnuts, toasted and chopped
2 tbsp chopped mint
2 tbsp chopped parsley

300g halloumi cheese, cut into slices
a few handfuls of rocket leaves to serve

Method

1. Heat 1 tbsp of the olive oil in a pan and sauté the onion and yellow pepper for 5–6 minutes, until starting to soften.
2. Add the garlic and cook for 1 minute. Remove from the heat and stir in the lentils.
3. Whisk together the remaining olive oil, balsamic vinegar, mustard and honey and toss the dressing through the lentils along with the pomegranate seeds, walnuts, mint and parsley.
4. Heat a griddle to hot and cook the slices of halloumi for 2–3 minutes on each side, until golden.
5. Serve the lentils on a bed of rocket leaves, topped with halloumi slices.

SMOKED HADDOCK AND POTATO CHOWDER

Serves 4

Ingredients

500g un-dyed smoked haddock fillet
600ml fish stock
6 peppercorns
2 bay leaves
60g butter
1 leek, trimmed and thinly sliced
25g gluten-free flour
500g potatoes, peeled and diced
600ml milk
100ml double cream
2 tbsp chopped parsley

Method

1. Place the haddock in a pan with the fish stock, peppercorns and bay leaves. Bring to a simmer and cook for 2–3 minutes, take off the heat and leave to cool for 5 minutes.
2. Drain the fish, reserving the stock and discarding the peppercorns and bay leaves.
3. Break the fish into large flakes.
4. Melt the butter in a large pan and sauté the leek for 5 minutes until tender.
5. Stir in the flour and cook for 1 minute before adding the reserved fish stock and bringing to the boil, stirring.
6. Add the potatoes, cover and simmer for 12–15 minutes until the potatoes are tender.
7. Stir in the milk and cream and bring back to a simmer. Stir in the haddock and half the parsley.
8. Pour into warmed bowls and sprinkle with the remaining parsley to serve.

THAI FISHCAKES WITH MANGO SALSA

Serves 4

Ingredients

500g cod loin fillet
100g cooked prawns
2 tbsp chopped coriander
3 spring onions, trimmed and finely sliced
2 tbsp Thai red curry paste
1 green chilli, deseeded and chopped
2 tbsp lime juice
1 mango, peeled, destoned and diced
1 small red onion, peeled and diced
¼ cucumber, diced
2 tbsp sunflower oil

Method

1. Place the cod and prawns in a food processor with 1 tbsp of the coriander, spring onions, curry paste, green chilli and 1 tbsp of lime juice and blend until the mixture is finely minced, but not smooth.
2. Form the mixture into walnut-sized balls then flatten them slightly (you should make approx. 16 fishcakes).
3. Place on a plate or board, cover and chill for 30 minutes.
4. Meanwhile, make the salsa by mixing together the mango, red onion, cucumber and remaining coriander and lime juice. Leave to stand at room temperature while you cook the fishcakes.
5. Heat the sunflower oil in a frying pan then add the fishcakes (you may need to do this in batches), cooking for 1–2 minutes on each side, until golden.
6. Serve with the mango salsa.

VIETNAMESE PRAWN AND RICE NOODLES

Serves 4

Ingredients

200g rice noodles
zest and juice of 1 orange
2 tbsp red curry paste
2 tsp fish sauce
2 tsp light brown soft sugar
2 tsp soy sauce
1 tbsp coconut oil
2cm piece fresh root ginger, peeled and diced
2 garlic cloves, peeled and sliced
1 stalk lemon grass, outer layers removed, and sliced
2 red peppers, deseeded and sliced
150g mangetout, shredded
125g beansprouts
350g raw king prawns

handful basil, chopped
handful coriander, chopped
2 tbsp salted peanuts, chopped

Method

1. Prepare the rice according to the pack instructions.
2. Mix together the orange zest and juice, curry paste, fish sauce, sugar, soy sauce and 2 tbsp water.
3. Heat the oil in a frying pan or wok and cook the ginger, garlic and lemon grass for 1 minute. Add the peppers and stir-fry for 2–3 minutes.
4. Toss in the shredded mangetout then pour in the previously made sauce.
5. Add the beansprouts and prawns and continue to stir-fry until the prawns are cooked through (have turned pink).
6. Drain the noodles and add them to the wok along with the chopped herbs. Toss together well.
7. Serve in warmed bowls, sprinkled with the chopped peanuts.

ALMOND CRUSTED SALMON WITH SPICY SWEET POTATO WEDGES

Serves 4

Ingredients

650g sweet potatoes, cut into wedges
2 tbsp olive oil
½ tsp smoked paprika
1 tsp freshly milled black pepper
4 salmon fillets
juice of 1 lemon
75g blanched almonds, finely chopped
1 tsp cumin seeds
½ tsp garam masala
2 tbsp chopped parsley

Method

1. Preheat the oven to 200°C (400°F) Gas mark 6.
2. Place the sweet potato wedges into a roasting tin and toss with the olive oil, paprika and pepper. Roast for 25–30 minutes, until soft.
3. Meanwhile, place the salmon fillets on a large piece of foil on a baking tray. Squeeze over the lemon juice.
4. Mix together the chopped almonds, cumin seeds and garam masala and sprinkle over the fillets. Wrap the fillets in the foil, bringing edges together to seal. Bake for 15 minutes.
5. Remove potatoes and salmon from the oven. Toss the chopped parsley through the sweet potatoes and serve with the salmon fillets.

CHICKEN AND CHICKPEA CURRY

Serves 4

Ingredients

2 tsp coconut oil
1 onion, peeled and chopped
1 red pepper, deseeded and thickly sliced
1–2 tbsp Thai red curry paste (or more if you like it hotter!)
350g chicken breast, cut into cubes
1 x 400g can coconut milk
1 x 400g can chickpeas, drained
175g baby spinach leaves
2 tbsp chopped coriander
basmati rice, cooked, to serve

Method

1. Heat the oil in a pan and cook the onion and red pepper for 4–5 minutes, until starting to soften.
2. Stir in the curry paste and cook for 1 minute before stirring in the chicken pieces. Stir well to coat with the curry sauce and cook for 6–8 minutes.

3. Pour in the coconut milk, bring to a simmer and cook for 12–15 minutes.
4. Stir in the chickpeas and spinach, cook for a further 2–3 minutes and then serve, sprinkled with chopped coriander and with rice if wished.

CHILLI CON CARNE

Serves 4

Ingredients

1 tbsp olive oil
1 onion, peeled and diced
1 red pepper, peeled and diced
2 garlic cloves, peeled and diced
2 tsp mild chilli powder
1 tsp smoked paprika
500g minced beef
300ml beef stock
1 x 400g can chopped tomatoes
2 tbsp tomato puree
1 tsp sugar
1 x 410g can kidney beans, drained
basmati rice, cooked, to serve
soured cream to serve

Method

1. Heat the oil in a large pan and sauté the onion and red pepper for 3–4 minutes.
2. Add the garlic and spices, stir well and cook for another 2–3 minutes.
3. Add the minced beef and cook to brown the meat all over, stirring from time to time.

4. Pour in the stock and chopped tomatoes along with the tomato puree and sugar.
5. Stir well and bring to a simmer, cover and cook for 20 minutes, stirring occasionally.
6. Add the drained beans and cook, uncovered, for another 10 minutes, adding a little water if needed.
7. Serve with basmati rice and a dollop of soured cream.

GLUTEN-FREE TOMATO AND ROCKET PIZZA

Serves 4 (makes 2 pizzas)

Ingredients

500g gluten-free flour
1 tsp salt
2 tsp quick yeast
2 tbsp caster sugar
300ml milk
4 tbsp olive oil
2 eggs, beaten
1 x 400g can chopped tomatoes
12 cherry tomatoes, halved
250g mozzarella, sliced
handful basil leaves, torn
large handful rocket leaves

Method

1. Preheat the oven to 180°C (350°F) Gas mark 4. Grease two baking sheets.
2. Mix together the flour, salt, yeast and sugar.
3. In a jug, whisk together the milk, oil and eggs.
4. Gradually add the wet ingredients to the dry and bring together to form a sticky dough.
5. Divide the dough in half and roll out both pieces to form a circle. Place each circle of dough on a greased baking tray. Leave to rise for 30 minutes.

6. Bake for 10–15 minutes, then remove from the oven and add the topping.
7. Spread with chopped tomatoes, and then top with the cherry tomatoes, mozzarella slices and torn basil leaves.
8. Bake for 35–40 minutes, until the base is crisp and the top is melted and golden.
9. Serve each one with a handful of rocket leaves sprinkled over the top.

GRIDDLED LAMB CHOPS WITH MINT & FETA MASH

Serves 4

Ingredients

4 lamb chops
2 garlic cloves, peeled and finely chopped
4 sprigs thyme, leaves only
1 tbsp olive oil
750g potatoes, peeled and chopped
200g frozen peas
60g butter
150ml milk
2 tbsp chopped mint
125g feta, crumbled
seasoning
steamed greens to serve (optional)

Method

1. Place the lamb chops in a non-metallic bowl and mix with the garlic, thyme and olive oil. Leave to marinate for 10–15 minutes.
2. Meanwhile, cook the potatoes in a pan of boiling water for 8–10 minutes, until they are tender, adding the peas for the last 2 minutes of cooking.

3. Heat a griddle and cook the lamb chops for 5–6 minutes on each side, depending on how pink you like your lamb.
4. Drain the potatoes and peas, and mash with the butter and milk, then stir in the mint and crumbled feta. Season to taste.
5. Serve the lamb chops with the minted mash, and steamed greens if desired.

MOROCCAN SEAFOOD TAGINE

Serves 4

Ingredients

1 tbsp olive oil
1 red onion, peeled and chopped
1 garlic clove, peeled and diced
1 red pepper, deseeded and chopped
2 tbsp harissa paste
2 x 400g cans chopped tomatoes
1 x 400g can chickpeas
100g squid, cleaned and cut into bite-size pieces
200g prawns
100g cod loin, cut into bite-size pieces
juice of ½ lemon
seasoning
small handful coriander leaves
2 tbsp flaked almonds, toasted
cooked quinoa or rice to serve

Method

1. Heat the oil in a large pan and sauté the onion, garlic and pepper for 3–4 minutes, until starting to soften.
2. Stir in the harissa paste, chopped tomatoes and chickpeas, and cook for 8–10 minutes.

3. Stir in the seafood and lemon juice and cook for 10–12 minutes, until the seafood is cooked.
4. Season to taste and stir in the coriander leaves and flaked almonds.
5. Serve with quinoa or rice if wished.

PAN-FRIED LEMON COD WITH PESTO CRUSHED POTATOES

Serves 4

Ingredients

zest and juice of 2 lemons
freshly milled black pepper
4 x 150g cod loins
750g potatoes, peeled and chopped
3 tbsp olive oil
2 tbsp pesto
2 large handfuls spinach leaves
seasoning
4 spring onions, trimmed and sliced

Method

1. Sprinkle the lemon zest, juice of 1 lemon and pepper over the cod loins and leave to stand for 12–15 minutes.
2. Cook the potatoes in a pan of boiling water for 12–15 minutes, until tender. Drain and return to the pan.
3. Heat 1 tbsp olive oil in a frying pan and cook the cod loins for 2 minutes on each side, until cooked through.
4. Meanwhile, crush the potatoes with a fork then mix in the remaining olive oil, lemon juice, pesto and spinach. Season to taste.
5. Serve the cod loins on a bed of crushed potatoes, sprinkled with sliced spring onion.

SESAME TUNA WITH CUCUMBER SALAD

Serves 4

Ingredients

1 large cucumber, peeled
1 tsp caster sugar
1 tbsp rice wine vinegar
100g sesame seeds
2 tsp freshly milled black pepper
4 tuna fillets
1 tbsp olive oil
1 tbsp soy sauce
1 tbsp sesame oil
2cm piece fresh root ginger, grated
1 garlic clove, crushed
1 red chilli, deseeded and sliced
2 spring onions, finely sliced
handful coriander leaves

Method

1. Slice the cucumber in half lengthways and, using a teaspoon, scoop out the seeds and discard. Cut into thick diagonal chunks and place in a bowl.
2. Add the sugar and vinegar and chill for 20 minutes.
3. Mix together the sesame seeds and freshly milled black pepper and place on a plate. Coat each of the tuna steaks in the sesame seeds.
4. Heat the olive oil in a griddle or frying pan and cook the tuna steaks for 4–5 minutes on each side, depending on how rare you like your tuna.
5. Add the remaining ingredients to the salad and serve with the tuna steaks.

KALE AND MACKEREL SALAD

Serves 4

Ingredients

4 eggs
2 tbsp tahini
4 tbsp extra virgin olive oil
2 tbsp balsamic vinegar
1 garlic clove, crushed
1 tsp honey
2 tbsp sunflower seeds
2 tbsp pumpkin seeds
2 tbsp sesame seeds
175g kale, shredded
2 carrots, peeled and grated
1 red pepper, deseeded and sliced
1 yellow pepper, deseeded and sliced
1 small red onion, peeled and thinly sliced
8 dried apricots, diced
4 smoked mackerel fillets, broken into large chunks
handful parsley, roughly chopped
handful mint, roughly chopped
handful coriander, roughly chopped

Method

1. Softly boil the eggs in a small pan of boiling water for 4–5 minutes, and then refresh under cold running water for 1 minute. Leave to cool before peeling off the shell and cutting in half.
2. Whisk together the tahini, olive oil, balsamic, garlic and honey.
3. Toast the sunflower, pumpkin and sesame seeds together in a dry pan, until they just start to change colour.
4. In a large salad bowl, toss together the kale, grated carrot, peppers, onion, apricots, mackerel and herbs.
5. Top with the eggs and then sprinkle over the seeds, and finally, the dressing.

TURKEY AND KIDNEY BEAN BURGERS WITH RED PEPPER SALSA

Serves 4

Ingredients

For the burgers

2 tbsp olive oil
1 tsp cumin seeds
1 onion, peeled and diced
1 garlic clove, crushed
500g turkey mince
1 x 210g can kidney beans, drained and roughly mashed
2 tbsp chopped coriander
seasoning

For the salsa

1 red pepper, deseeded and diced
1 small red onion, peeled and diced
2 tomatoes, diced
2 tbsp chopped parsley
½ tbsp balsamic vinegar

crunchy green salad to serve

Method

1. Heat half the oil in a frying pan with the cumin seeds, then add the onion and garlic and cook for 3–4 minutes, until the onion starts to soften.
2. Place in a bowl with the remaining burger ingredients and mix really well.
3. Shape into four burgers and chill while you make the salsa.
4. Mix all the salsa ingredients together and leave to stand at room temperature while you cook the burgers.
5. Heat the remaining oil in the frying pan and cook the burgers for 7–8 minutes on either side, until cooked through.
6. Serve on a crunchy green salad, with the salsa spooned over.

BANANA AND STRAWBERRY MUFFINS

Makes 8

Ingredients

300g gluten-free flour
2 tsp gluten-free baking powder
75g soft dark brown sugar
2 bananas, peeled and chopped
juice of 1 lemon
75g coconut oil, melted
100ml milk
75g strawberries, hulled and chopped

Method

1. Preheat the oven to 175°C (325°F) Gas mark 3. Line a muffin tin with 8 paper cases.
2. Place the flour, baking powder and sugar in a bowl and mix well.
3. Mash the banana with the lemon juice.
4. Mix together the coconut oil, milk and beaten egg.
5. Pour the coconut oil mixture into the flour and mix together just a little.
6. Gently stir in the banana and strawberries – do not over mix.
7. Spoon into the paper cases and bake in the oven for 25 minutes, until golden.

FLORENTINES

Makes 12

Ingredients

50g unsalted butter
100g caster sugar
50ml thick double cream
175g flaked almonds
15g mixed peel, diced
10g currants
1 egg white
100g dark chocolate, melted

Method

1. Preheat the oven to 180°C (350°F) Gas mark 4. Line two baking sheets with baking paper.
2. Place the butter and sugar in a small pan with 2 tbsp water. Bring to the boil then cook on a high heat for 5 minutes, until the mixture starts to become pale. Remove from the heat and leave to cool for 2 minutes.
3. Stir in the cream, almonds, mixed peel and currants.
4. Whisk the egg white to soft peaks then gently fold into the fruit and nut mixture.
5. Spoon the mixture onto the prepared baking sheets to make 12 florentines, leaving space between each one.
6. Bake for 15–18 minutes, until golden. Carefully slide onto a cooling rack and leave to cool.
7. Spread the bottom of each Florentine with melted dark chocolate and leave to set.

LEMON DRIZZLE CAKE

Serves 8–10

Ingredients

175g unsalted butter
zest and juice of 2 lemons
175g caster sugar
2 large eggs, lightly beaten
175g gluten-free self-raising flour
1 tbsp poppy seeds
3 tbsp icing sugar

Method

1. Preheat the oven to 180°C (375°F) Gas mark 4. Grease and base line an 18cm loaf tin.
2. Cream together the butter, lemon zest and sugar, until light and fluffy.
3. Beat in the eggs, a little at a time, adding a little flour if the mixture starts to curdle.
4. Fold in the remaining flour along with the poppy seeds and 1 tbsp lemon juice.
5. Spoon the mixture into the tin and level the top.
6. Bake for 40–45 minutes, until a sharp knife inserted into the centre comes out clean.
7. Remove from the oven and allow to cool slightly, then remove from the tin and cool on a cooling rack.
8. Mix together the remaining lemon juice and icing sugar and spoon over the cake, allowing it to drizzle down the sides (you may need to spread it with a warmed knife).
9. Serve cut into slices.

ORANGE POLENTA CAKE

Serves 6–8

Ingredients

200g unsalted butter
200g caster sugar
200g ground almonds
100g fine polenta
1½ tsp gluten-free baking powder
3 large eggs, lightly beaten
zest and juice of 2 small oranges
125g icing sugar
natural yoghurt to serve (optional)

Method

1. Preheat the oven to 180°C (350°F) Gas mark 4. Grease and base line a 23cm spring-form cake tin.
2. Cream together the butter and sugar until pale and light in texture.
3. Mix together the ground almonds, polenta and baking powder then mix a little into the butter mixture, along with a little beaten egg. Continue to add almond mixture and eggs alternately until all combined.
4. Beat in the orange zest and then spoon the mixture into the prepared tin. Bake for 35–40 minutes, until a skewer inserted into the centre comes out clean. Leave to cool in the tin.
5. Meanwhile, place the orange juice and icing sugar in a small pan and bring to the boil. Once the icing sugar is dissolved, remove from the heat and leave to cool slightly.
6. Prick the cake all over with a cocktail stick then pour the syrup over the cake. Leave to cool completely before removing the cake from the tin.
7. Serve cut into wedges with a dollop of natural yoghurt if wished.

WELSH CAKES

Makes 16

Ingredients

350g gluten-free flour
1 tsp gluten-free baking powder
¼ tsp mixed spice
150g unsalted butter
100g caster sugar
grated zest of 1 orange
100g mixed dried fruit
2 eggs, lightly beaten
2 tsp coconut oil, melted
1 tsp lemon juice

Method

1. Sift the flour, baking powder and mixed spice into a large bowl.
2. Rub the butter into the flour mixture using your fingertips.
3. Stir in the sugar, orange zest and dried fruit.
4. Stir in the beaten egg, oil and lemon juice and bring together to make a soft dough.
5. Turn out onto a floured work surface and roll to approx 5mm thickness. Cut with biscuit cutter into 3–4cm circles.
6. Cook on a hot griddle or in a hot frying pan, for 2–3 minutes on each side, until golden.

Acknowledgements

I cannot finish without acknowledging all the support of my wonderful colleagues (consultants, research fellows, secretaries, nurses and medical students) over the years who have encouraged me and guided me and looked after me.

My loving family in Sheffield, Edinburgh and London, they are the best part of me.

Finally, I would like to offer a heartfelt thanks to the people and patients of Sheffield (and in particular the regional and national Coeliac UK group) who have been so generous with their time and both supported and taken part in so many studies over the years.

If you are interested in learning more about what we do or would like to support our work or make a donation towards this research please look at our charity website: www.thebret.org

Glossary

Anaemia: A reduction in the number of red blood cells or haemoglobin in our blood. Forms of anaemia can be related to iron deficiency, low vitamin B12 or folate.

Atopic Diseases: Diseases of an allergic origin such as asthma, eczema, urticaria and hay fever.

Autoimmune Disease: A condition caused by the body's immune system attacking itself.

Bile Acid Malabsorption: Sometimes also called bile acid diarrhoea and associated to many gut diseases and may present with chronic diarrhoea.

Duodenal Biopsy: A snip of human tissue (biopsy) taken from the lining of the small bowel. The first part of the small bowel beyond the stomach is called the duodenum.

Enteropathy: Another term for damage of the small bowel. If termed gluten sensitive enteropathy then this is another term for coeliac disease.

Exocrine Pancreatic Insufficiency: The pancreas has two gland systems, the endocrine system involved in producing things like insulin and the exocrine system which produces digestive enzymes. Exocrine pancreatic insufficiency is an inability to produce these digestive enzymes or a reduction in production.

Fibromyalgia: A long-term condition which causes muscular or musculoskeletal pain with stiffness and tenderness at localised points in the body.

Gastroscopy: A flexible endoscope or camera which is passed into our mouth and down the upper part of our digestive system.

HLA: This is a genetic profile which is described as HLADQ2 or DQ8 (Human Leucocyte Antigen). We all have HLA genes but there is a particular HLA code that associates itself with coeliac disease. Virtually everyone who has coeliac disease has this specific HLADQ2 or DQ8 gene code.

Irritable Bowel Syndrome: Is not a disease but a syndrome. It is a chronic condition affecting some individuals' digestive systems. It presents with bloating, abdominal discomfort or pain and may have associated diarrhoea or constipation.

Isotope: A variant of a particular chemical element which differs in neutron numbers. Isotopes can allow us to measure the chemical composition or determine the age of geological objects.

Malabsorption: A problem with absorption. The intestine cannot absorb nutrients (proteins, carbohydrates and fats) across the bowel and into our blood stream.

Malnutrition: A condition that results in eating a diet in which the nutrients are not enough to sustain us. This is frequently associated with weight loss.

Nocebo: This is the opposite if you wish of the placebo effect. In the placebo effect you think an inert intervention is benefiting you. In the nocebo effect you think an intervention is causing you harm.

Placebo: In drug study terms is essentially something participants can be given which is inert or harmless. The reason for doing this is that participants can be influenced in a positive way by such an inert intervention.

Prevalence: In medical terms is the number of people affected by a disease at a particular time.

Probiotics: Live bacteria and yeasts that may have a beneficial effect on our health and digestive system.

Rome Criteria: A classification system for describing IBS. This is based on the meeting of an international consensus group who originally met in Rome. Any further iterations of this consensus are called Rome II, or Rome III.

Serological Test: A blood test looking for specific markers, for example in coeliac disease it is the presence of antibodies.

Small Bowel Bacterial Overgrowth: The presence of excess bacteria in the small bowel which may be harmful and cause symptoms such as diarrhoea.

T-Cell: A cell within our immune system. This is a type of white blood cell (also sometimes known as T-lymphocyte) that is involved in the defence of our body.

Villous Atrophy: A loss of the lining of the normal small bowel. The normal small bowel has finger-like projections when looked at down a microscope. These are called villi. If these villi are damaged then the term for this is 'atrophy'. Villous atrophy is a crucial part of coeliac disease.

FODMAP Food List

The Low FODMAP Diet

The low FODMAP diet involves *two* phases. High FODMAP foods should be avoided for 2 to 6 weeks. It is recommended that a dietitian with experience in this approach should then be consulted to help guide reintroduction to tolerance of FODMAP containing foods. This helps tailor the diet to the individual, increases variety and nutritional balance.

Please note fresh meats, fish, poultry, tofu, and plain quorn are low FODMAP foods as are butter, margarines and oils so can be eaten freely, within the context of 'Healthy eating' guidelines.

Foods listed 'In Moderation' or with a stated portion size should be limited to one portion per meal or snack.

Cereals:

Food Group	Suitable Foods	In Moderation	Foods To Avoid
Grains and Starchy Vegetables	Buckwheat, polenta, quinoa, rice, corn (maize), millet, potato (plain salted crisps), yams, plantain, ackee, sorghum, tapioca (and flours of the above)	Sweet potato (70g/2.5oz), cassava (70g/2.5oz)	Wheat, wheat-bran, barely, bulghar wheat, rye, couscous, amaranth
Breads	Wheat or gluten free breads (rice, oat, corn, potato, sorghum, tapioca flour based) 100% sourdough spelt-bread		Wheat, barely, rye based breads and rolls including white, brown, granary, pitta bread, bagels, panini, naan, pizza bases etc.

Food Group	Suitable Foods	In Moderation	Foods To Avoid
Flours	Wheat-free or gluten free flour, cornflour, maize flour, potato flour, polenta, pounded yam, rice flour, sorghum flour, baking powder, bicarbonate of soda, cream of tartar		All wheat flours (white, plain, self raising, wholemeal), rye flour, barley flour, spelt flour, soya flour
Cakes and Biscuits	Gluten free biscuits and crackers, oatcakes, rice-cakes, flapjacks, flourless cakes, (check ingredients for fructose, sorbitol, dried fruit, or onion and garlic if savory)	Corn-cakes (24g/0.5 oz).	Wheat, barley, rye based cakes and biscuits i.e. water biscuits, crisp-breads, wheat crackers, rye crisp-breads, cream crackers, spelt crackers
Pasta and Noodles	Gluten free pasta and noodles, rice noodles, 100% buckwheat pasta, quinoa pasta		Wheat based noodles and pasta, spelt pasta, gnocchi
Breakfast Cereals	Porridge, oats, oatmeal, gluten free cornflakes and crisped rice, rice flakes, quinoa flakes (check ingredients for fructose, honey)	Cornflakes (30g/1oz), crisped-rice (30g/1oz)	Wheat, rye, barley and spelt based breakfast cereals, granola, muesli, honey containing cereals

Fruits:

Food Group	Suitable Foods	In Moderation	Foods To Avoid
Fruit: (Fresh, Dried, Juice) Limit portion size of suitable foods or foods in moderation to one portion per snack/meal. Portion size = Fresh fruit 80g. Fruit juice 100mls. Dried Fruit (see list).	Banana (1), blueberry (small bowl), breadfruit (1), honeydew melon (1 slice), cantaloupe melon (1 slice), carambola/ starfruit (1), clementine (2), cranberries (small bowl), dragonfruit (1), durian (1), grapes (10), kiwifruit (2), lemon (juice of 1), lime (juice of 1), mandarin (1-2), orange (1), papaya/paw paw (1 slice), pineapple (1 slice), raspberry (small bowl), rhubarb (small bowl), strawberry (small bowl).	Dried banana (20g/0.7oz), dried coconut (20g/0.7oz), dried cranberries (15g/0.5oz), dried currants (15g/0.5oz), raisins (15g/0.5oz).	Apples, apricots, avocado, blackberry, cherries, currants, dates, figs (dried/ fresh), grapefruit, goji berries, lychee, mango, nectarine, peach, pear, plum, prunes, pomegranate, tamarillo, watermelon. Tinned fruit in apple or pear juice.

Vegetables:

Food Group	Suitable Foods	In Moderation	Foods To Avoid
Vegetables Limit portion size of 'In Moderation' foods to one portion per snack/meal.	Alfalfa, aubergine, beansprouts, green beans, bell peppers, bok choy, brussels sprouts, cabbage (white and red), carrot, celeriac, chilli (green and red), chives, choy sum, collard greens, courgette, cucumber, fennel, ginger root, kale, lettuce, rocket, okra, spring onion (green tops only), parsnips, potato, radish, spinach, tomato, turnip, water chestnuts	Broccoli (50g/1.7oz), butternut squash (30g/1oz), sweet-corn (40g/1.4oz), chana dal boiled (40g/1.4oz), chickpeas canned (40g/1.4oz), lentils canned (40g/1.4oz), urid dal boiled (40g/1.4oz)	Artichoke, asparagus, all beans and pulses (except beans in moderate section), beetroot, savoy cabbage, cauliflower, celery, garlic, leek, mange tout, mushroom, onion, sugar snap peas, peas

Nuts/Seeds:

Food Group	Suitable Foods	In Moderation	Foods To Avoid
Nuts / Seeds Limit portion size of 'In Moderation' foods to one portion per snack/meal.	Chestnuts, linseed (flax), macadamia, brazil, peanuts, pecan, pine nuts, chia seeds, poppy seeds, pumpkin seeds, sesame seeds, sunflower seeds, walnuts	Almonds (12g – 10 nuts), hazelnuts (12g – 10 nuts)	Cashews, pistachios

Milk and Dairy:

Food Group	Suitable Foods	In Moderation	Foods To Avoid
Milk and Dairy Limit portion size of 'In Moderation' foods to one portion per snack/meal. Milk alternative products may contain added FODMAPs, such as apple juice, FOS, inulin, therefore you should check the ingredients label	Lactose free milk/yoghurt, almond milk, hemp milk, soya milk, (unsweetened), cheddar, camembert, feta, goats cheese, mozzarella, pecorino, brie, whipped cream, soya yoghurt, soya custard and soya custard desserts, soya ice cream, dark chocolate (check flavorings)	Cottage cheese (35g/1.2oz) Haloumi (50g/1.7oz) Ricotta (40g/1.4oz)	Milk (whole, semi-skimmed, skimmed), buttermilk, yoghurts (including greek, drinking and diet varieties), rice milk, oat milk, coconut milk, custard, ice cream, processed cheese, cheese slices, reduced fat cheese, quark, low fat soft cheese, malted milk drinks e.g. horlicks, bournvita, ovaltine, milo, options, drinking chocolate buttermilk, milk chocolate

Drinks:

Food Group	Suitable Foods	In Moderation	Foods To Avoid
Soft Drinks	Take 6-8 glasses (1.5 - 2 liters) of fluid per day. Try to choose water and non-caffeinated drinks such as peppermint tea, green tea, dilute squash	Fizzy drinks and caffeinated drinks can increase IBS symptoms in some people	Chai tea, chamomile tea, oolong tea, fennel tea, chicory (camp coffee), coconut water, dandelion tea, fennel tea, carob powder
Alcohol	Most alcoholic drinks (wine, beers, vodka, gin, whiskey) are low in FODMAPs but for some people alcohol may cause IBS symptoms. (If you do drink alcohol keep within suggested healthy limits).		Rum, dessert wine

Sugars and sweeteners:

Food Group	Suitable Foods	In Moderation	Foods To Avoid
Sugars and Sweeteners	Golden syrup, maple syrup, treacle, jam (made from suitable fruits in the suitable section above), marmalade (check for high FODMAP sweeteners), aspartame, acesulfame k, saccharin, candarel, silver spoon, splenda, hermesetas		Honey, agave nectar, fructose based sweeteners such as glucose-fructose syrup, fructose syrup, high fructose corn syrup Sorbitol, mannitol, lactilol, maltilol, xylitol, erthritol (may be added to mints, chewing gum, chocolate, sweets or drinks)

Added Ingredients:

Food Group	Suitable Foods	In Moderation	Foods To Avoid
Ingredients to look out for	Herbs and spices such as chilli, dried herbs, vinegar, pepper and salt, MSG, arrowroot, buckwheat flour, cornflour, millet flour, maize flour, polenta, baking powder, bicarbonate of soda, cream of tartar, yeast, garlic infused oil, spring onion (green part)		Garlic – powder, puree, extract, salt or dried onion – powder, puree, extract or dried FOS, inulin, solids, milk powder, milk protein, milk fat, whey, hydrolysed whey protein, hydrolyzed whey sugar, rennet, lactoalbumin, lactoglobulin, milk solids, lactose, casein, caseinates, hydrolysed casein

Index